diabetes management system

personal planner

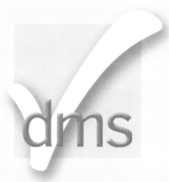

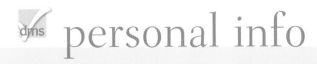

personal info

name _____ date _____

phone numbers **h)** _____ **w)** _____ **c)** _____

testing & numbers

last fasting blood glucose test _____ result _____

last A1c test _____ result _____

last cholesterol test _____

Total cholesterol _____

LDL cholesterol _____

HDL cholesterol _____

last blood pressure test _____ result _____

medications

Diabetes medications _____ dose_____

_____ dose_____

Other medications _____

_____

my contacts

doctor_____ ☏ _____

dietitian _____ ☏ _____

pharmacist_____ ☏ _____

emergency_____ ☏ _____

> "You are never too old to set another goal or to dream a new dream"
>
> — C. S. Lewis

personal contract

start date ✳

I vow to myself that over the next ten weeks I will eat, move, and choose to beat diabetes by following the principles of the DMS. I agree that I will:

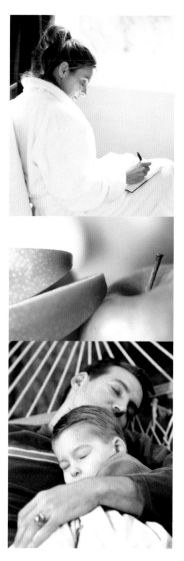

Track my weight and blood sugar daily *[Initial]*

Follow the weekly assignments in this planner *[Initial]*

Plan my meals every week *[Initial]*

Fill out the Daily Tracker every day *[Initial]*

Follow the DMS walking plan *[Initial]*

On the DMS I fully expect to:

☐ Lower my blood sugar

☐ Lose 5-10 percent of my body weight over 6 months

☐ Increase my insulin sensitivity and perhaps lower my dose of insulin or diabetes medication, with my doctor's okay

I agree to look at this contract regularly to remind myself of my commitment.

signed

witnessed by

12 golden rules to eat to beat diabetes

Good news! Eating to manage diabetes is easier than ever. Nutritionists now know that people with diabetes don't have to completely shun sugar. It's total calories that count most, no matter where those calories come from. Carbs aren't all bad—the goal is to choose the right carbs. And believe it or not, the "good" fats are actually good for your diabetes! Follow these 12 rules and you'll be well on your way to success.

1 Eat more often. Eating small meals and healthy snacks throughout the day will help you avoid blood sugar swings and keep your metabolism revved up so you burn more calories all day. Always eat breakfast, and never go more than four hours without a small meal or snack.

2 Be smart about snacks. Snacking is smart, but keep snacks to under 150 calories, and favor fruits, nuts, raw vegetables, and yogurt over chips and cookies.

3 Hail the whole. Unlike simple carbs, complex carbs such as whole grains are "slow burning," so their impact on blood sugar is gentler. Give preference to whole grain bread, whole wheat pasta, and brown rice.

4 Avoid "white" foods. "Simple" or "refined" carbs, such as table sugar, white bread, and cereals made primarily from rice or corn, are digested quickly. In no time, they're broken down into glucose, which sends your blood sugar soaring. In turn, your body pumps out more insulin, and when all that insulin kicks in, blood sugar plummets, leaving you shaky and hungry again.

5 Eat outside the box. Packaged foods are often high in fat, calories, and heart-damaging hydrogenated oils. Whenever you can, cook your own meals from fresh foods instead.

6 Avoid sugary drinks. Each 12-ounce serving of regular soda contains about 150 calories—virtually all of it sugar. And studies show that soda calories don't fill you up the way food does, so you end up consuming more calories throughout the day than you would if you got those 150 calories from food. Choose water, skim milk, or unsweetened tea.

7 Fill up on fiber. It slows digestion and keeps blood sugar from rising quickly after a meal. It adds bulk to food, so it makes you feel full without adding calories. Vegetables and beans are great sources.

8 Eat protein at every meal. This is critical because protein makes you feel full longer than carbohydrates do. Protein also has the advantage of being digested more slowly than carbohydrates, so it doesn't have the dramatic impact on blood sugar that carbs do.

9 Choose lean protein. Fatty steaks and hamburgers are not the answer to diabetes. They're high in saturated fat, which clogs arteries that are already vulnerable to heart disease and makes cells more resistant to insulin. Choose meats that are relatively low in saturated fat: skinless chicken breast, top round, sirloin, and tenderloin. Fish is another good choice.

10 Fill half your plate with vegetables. When you do, you'll automatically eat fewer starches and less fat—and that means fewer calories.

11 Favor good fats. Unlike saturated fats, unsaturated fats are actually good for you. Monounsaturated fats even help reduce insulin resistance and make blood sugar easier to control. Get it in olive and canola oil, almonds and other nuts, avocados, peanuts, and peanut butter.

12 Dine on dairy. Consuming more milk, yogurt, and other dairy foods may actually help you lose weight. The reason: A lack of adequate calcium triggers the release of a hormone called calcitriol, which prompts the body to store fat. Eating two or three servings of calcium-rich dairy foods per day helps keep calcitriol levels low so your body burns more fat and stores less. Choose low-fat or nonfat dairy foods.

walking

for better diabetes control

Get out the door today and find your stride again! Most of us no longer need to hoof it to get where we're going, so dedicate time for walking around your neighborhood or a pretty walking trail. Why? Exercise increases your cells' sensitivity to insulin, which allows them to soak up more glucose, lowering your blood sugar level. That makes it one of the best things you can do to control diabetes. It could even help you get off insulin or diabetes medication, or at least lower your dose. It's also an effective way to trim fat from your body and slash your risk of a heart attack.

Starting today, we want you to lace up a good pair of sneakers and walk three times a week, building up to five times a week. Start as slowly as you like. Gradually you'll pick up the pace and add to the length of your walks, so that by Week 10 you'll be working your heart and muscles enough to really make a difference. Keep track of your walking on the Daily Tracker pages of this planner.

To encourage yourself to walk more, consider buying a pedometer, a small gadget that counts your steps. If you do, log your steps on the Daily Tracker. Aim for a goal of 50,000 steps a week.

To avoid hypoglycemia—if you take insulin or diabetes medication—time your workout so that you're not exercising when the insulin or drug activity peaks. For the same reason, exercise after a meal or a snack. Don't exercise if your blood sugar is below 100 mg/dl. If you start to feel shaky or light-headed during your walk, stop walking and have a small high-carb snack (carry one with you) such as 10 small jellybeans.

plan

10 Week Routine

			per week
week one	**15** MINUTES	Walk at whatever pace feels comfortable. Getting out the door is the goal.	3-5 times
week two	**20** MINUTES	Still comfortable	3-5 times
week three		Start cranking up the intensity a bit	5 times
week four	**25** MINUTES	You should be breathing hard but still able to hold a conversation	5 times
week five		Breathing hard	
week six	**30** MINUTES	Breathing hard	5 times
week seven		Breathing hard	
week eight	**35** MINUTES	Breathing hard	5 times
week nine		Breathing hard	
week ten	**40** MINUTES	Seek hills or walk on sand to make your workout more challenging	5 times

dms weekly meal planner

	Monday	Tuesday	Wednesday
breakfast			
lunch			
dinner			

The key to healthy eating is planning ahead. Plotting your dinners is most important. The trick is to find 8 or 10 healthy recipes you love (you may even want to keep a list on your refrigerator), then rotate them in.

If you don't mind leftovers, make extra and serve leftovers, either for lunch or dinner, at least once or twice a week. If you're planning to take leftovers for lunch, store them in single-serving containers so your lunch is ready to go when you are.

For other lunches, buy sliced turkey, whole wheat bread or rolls, and a bag of prewashed lettuce at the beginning of the week, and stock the pantry with cans of tuna fish and lentil or black bean soup.

	Thursday	Friday	Saturday	Sunday

Food Fact One cup of pearl barley (which doesn't require any soaking before cooking) has 10 grams of fiber, nearly half your daily target.

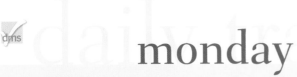

monday

my numbers

weight _____   blood sugar (time/level) _____ / _____ • _____ / _____ • _____ / _____ • _____ / _____

what I ate today

circle the number of servings

fruit

0 1 2 3 **4**

vegetables

0 1 2 3 4 **5**

whole grains

0 1 2 3 4 5 **6**

calcium-rich foods

0 1 **2 3**

beans

0 1 2

fish

0 1 2

extra lean poultry or meat

0 1 2

glasses of water

0 1 2 3 4 5 6 **7 8** 9 10

times I ate out of boredom, stress, or habit

0 1 2 3 4 5

※ Tip of the day - When you go for your walk, seek soft surfaces. Walking or jogging on hard surfaces such as concrete can be hard on the joints and the feet. Whenever possible, walk on grass, a dirt road, or a running track at the local high school or YMCA.

taking charge of my health!

eat

☐ ate a healthy breakfast

☐ had protein at every meal

☐ had 1-2 healthy snacks

☐ ate dinner by 7:00 p.m.

☐ avoided "white" foods

☐ drank water or tea instead of sugary drinks

move

☐ walked _____ steps/minutes

☐ made active choices

☐ got other exercise

_____

choose

☐ took my vitamins

☐ got enough sleep _____ hrs

☐ kept TV time under 2 hours

successes & confessions

rate your attitude today

3 excellent

2 good

1 so-so

0 disaster! plan to do better tomorrow

Try a new **vegetable** this week.

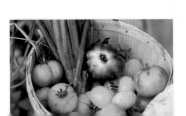

dfhs

tuesday

my numbers

weight _____   blood sugar (time/level) _____ / _____ • _____ / _____ • _____ / _____ • _____ / _____

✳ **Tip of the day** - Choose the lowest-fat meats and poultry. Chicken breast and pork loin are excellent choices. "Select" is the leanest grade of beef, followed by "choice" and "prime." Any meat with the word round (eye of round, top round, ground round) or loin (tenderloin, sirloin) is generally a leaner cut. When it's time to splurge, cook or order filet mignon— expensive, but lean.

taking charge of my health!

eat

- ☐ ate a healthy breakfast
- ☐ had protein at every meal
- ☐ had 1-2 healthy snacks
- ☐ ate dinner by 7:00 p.m.
- ☐ avoided "white" foods
- ☐ drank water or tea instead of sugary drinks

move

- ☐ walked _____ steps/minutes
- ☐ made active choices
- ☐ got other exercise

_____

choose

- ☐ took my vitamins
- ☐ got enough sleep _____ hrs
- ☐ kept TV time under 2 hours

successes & confessions

rate your attitude today

3   excellent
2   good
1   so-so
0   disaster! plan to do better tomorrow

did you **laugh** today?

what I ate today

circle the number of servings

fruit

0 1 2 3 **4**

vegetables

0 1 2 3 4 **5**

whole grains

0 1 2 3 4 5 **6**

calcium-rich foods

0 1 **2** **3**

beans

0 1 2

fish

0 1 2

extra lean poultry or meat

0 1 2

glasses of water

0 1 2 3 4 5 6 **7** **8** 9 10

times I ate out of boredom, stress, or habit

0 **1** 2 3 4 5

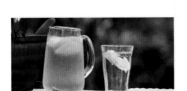

wednesday

my numbers

weight _____   blood sugar (time/level) _____ / _____ • _____ / _____ • _____ / _____ • _____ / _____

what I ate today

circle the number of servings

fruit

0 1 2 3 **4**

vegetables

0 1 2 3 4 **5**

whole grains

0 1 2 3 4 5 **6**

calcium-rich foods

0 1 **2** **3**

beans

0 1 2

fish

0 1 2

extra lean poultry or meat

0 1 2

glasses of water

0 1 2 3 4 5 6 **7** **8** 9 10

times I ate out of boredom, stress, or habit

0 **1** 2 3 4 5

✳ **Tip of the day** - For some people, exercise videos (or DVDs) are a terrific way to work in a workout. But before you buy one, try it. Many video rental stores have exercise videos for rent. "Test drive" a few different videos, then buy one you know you like. Choose tapes that describe the workout as "low intensity" or "low impact."

taking charge of my health!

eat

☐ ate a healthy breakfast

☐ had protein at every meal

☐ had 1-2 healthy snacks

☐ ate dinner by 7:00 p.m.

☐ avoided "white" foods

☐ drank water or tea instead of sugary drinks

move

☐ walked _____ steps/minutes

☐ made active choices

☐ got other exercise

_____

choose

☐ took my vitamins

☐ got enough sleep _____ hrs

☐ kept TV time under 2 hours

successes & confessions

rate your attitude today

3   excellent

2   good

1   so-so

0   disaster! plan to do better tomorrow

✳ Did you **drink enough water** today?

thursday

❋ Tip of the day - Believe that you can succeed. When it comes to weight loss, exercise, and just about any other challenge, truly believing that you can succeed will help you reach your goals. Build faith by setting very small goals at first—taking two short walks in a week, for example, or skipping dessert two nights in a row. As you succeed at achieving small goals, build on your successes.

taking charge of my health!

eat

☐ ate a healthy breakfast
☐ had protein at every meal
☐ had 1-2 healthy snacks
☐ ate dinner by 7:00 p.m.
☐ avoided "white" foods
☐ drank water or tea instead of sugary drinks

move

☐ walked _____ steps/minutes
☐ made active choices
☐ got other exercise

_____

choose

☐ took my vitamins
☐ got enough sleep _____ hrs
☐ kept TV time under 2 hours

successes & confessions

rate your attitude today

3 excellent
2 good
1 so-so
0 disaster! plan to do better tomorrow

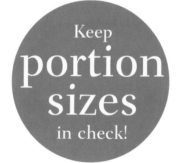

Keep **portion sizes** in check!

what I ate today

circle the number of servings

fruit

0 1 2 3 **4**

vegetables

0 1 2 3 4 **5**

whole grains

0 1 2 3 4 5 **6**

calcium-rich foods

0 1 **2 3**

beans

0 1 2

fish

0 1 2

extra lean poultry or meat

0 1 2

glasses of water

0 1 2 3 4 5 6 **7 8** 9 10

times I ate out of boredom, stress, or habit

0 1 2 3 4 5

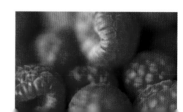

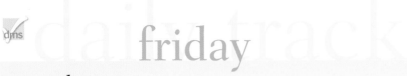

my numbers

weight _____   blood sugar (time/level) _____ / _____ • _____ / _____ • _____ / _____ • _____ / _____

what I ate today

circle the number of servings

fruit

0 1 2 3 **4**

vegetables

0 1 2 3 4 **5**

whole grains

0 1 2 3 4 5 **6**

calcium-rich foods

0 1 **2 3**

beans

0 1 2

fish

0 1 2

extra lean poultry or meat

0 1 2

glasses of water

0 1 2 3 4 5 6 **7 8** 9 10

times I ate out of boredom, stress, or habit

0 1 2 3 4 5

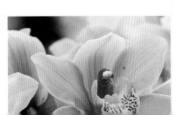

✳ **Tip of the day** - Make it easy to eat more fresh produce. For quick, nutrient-rich, low-calorie snacking throughout the week, wash, cut, and bag hardy fruits and vegetables such as cucumbers, zucchini, radishes, carrots, celery, cherry tomatoes, bell pepper slices, melon balls, grapes, and berries. The easier they are to grab, the more likely you'll be to eat them.

taking charge of my health!

eat

☐ ate a healthy breakfast
☐ had protein at every meal
☐ had 1-2 healthy snacks
☐ ate dinner by 7:00 p.m.
☐ avoided "white" foods
☐ drank water or tea instead of sugary drinks

move

☐ walked _____ steps/minutes
☐ made active choices
☐ got other exercise

_____

choose

☐ took my vitamins
☐ got enough sleep _____ hrs
☐ kept TV time under 2 hours

successes & confessions

rate your attitude today

3 excellent
2 good
1 so-so
0 disaster! plan to do better tomorrow

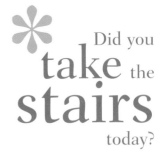

✳ Did you **take** the **stairs** today?

saturday

✳ Tip of the day - When you exercise, treat your feet well. People with diabetes are at an increased risk of skin infections, particularly in the feet. Make sure your sneakers fit properly and don't pinch. Wear cushiony socks. And check your feet after each exercise session for cuts, sores, blisters, ulcers, or redness.

what I ate today

circle the number of servings

fruit

0 1 2 3 **4**

vegetables

0 1 2 3 4 **5**

whole grains

0 1 2 3 4 5 **6**

calcium-rich foods

0 1 **2** 3

beans

0 1 2

fish

0 1 2

extra lean poultry or meat

0 1 2

glasses of water

0 1 2 3 4 5 6 **7** **8** 9 10

times I ate out of boredom, stress, or habit

0 **1** 2 3 4 5

taking charge of my health!

eat

☐ ate a healthy breakfast
☐ had protein at every meal
☐ had 1-2 healthy snacks
☐ ate dinner by 7:00 p.m.
☐ avoided "white" foods
☐ drank water or tea instead of sugary drinks

move

☐ walked _____ steps/minutes
☐ made active choices
☐ got other exercise
_____

choose

☐ took my vitamins
☐ got enough sleep _____ hrs
☐ kept TV time under 2 hours

successes & confessions

rate your attitude today

3 excellent
2 good
1 so-so
0 disaster! plan to do better tomorrow

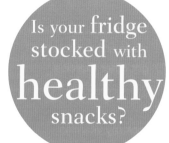

Is your fridge stocked with healthy snacks?

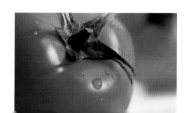

sunday

my numbers

weight _____   blood sugar (time/level) _____ / _____ • _____ / _____ • _____ / _____ • _____ / _____

what I ate today

circle the number of servings

fruit

0 1 2 3 **4**

vegetables

0 1 2 3 4 **5**

whole grains

0 1 2 3 4 5 **6**

calcium-rich foods

0 1 **2** 3

beans

0 1 2

fish

0 1 2

extra lean poultry or meat

0 1 2

glasses of water

0 1 2 3 4 5 6 **7** **8** 9 10

times I ate out of boredom, stress, or habit

0 **1** 2 3 4 5

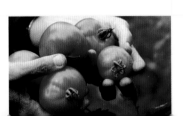

※ **Tip of the day** - Start the day with a high-fiber cereal. Fiber fills you up and keeps you full longer than sugary foods. Studies show that people who start the day with a high-fiber breakfast eat less later on. Look for a brand with at least 3 grams of fiber per serving. For a burst of flavor, add fresh fruit.

taking charge of my health!

eat

☐ ate a healthy breakfast
☐ had protein at every meal
☐ had 1-2 healthy snacks
☐ ate dinner by 7:00 p.m.
☐ avoided "white" foods
☐ drank water or tea instead of sugary drinks

move

☐ walked _____ steps/minutes
☐ made active choices
☐ got other exercise

_____

choose

☐ took my vitamins
☐ got enough sleep _____ hrs
☐ kept TV time under 2 hours

successes & confessions

rate your attitude today

3 excellent
2 good
1 so-so
0 disaster! plan to do better tomorrow

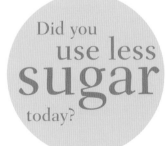

Did you **use less sugar** today?

week in review & ahead >

how well I did

eat

Improved my eating
from previous week   [Yes] [No]

Made healthy
restaurant choices   [Yes] [No]

Tried a new fruit,
vegetable, or grain   [Yes] [No]

move

Total walking time _____

Total steps _____
(if using a pedometer)

Walked more than
I did previous week   [Yes] [No]

Moved more than
I did previous week   [Yes] [No]

Felt more energized
than previous week   [Yes] [No]

choose

My attitude this week was:

☐ Positive—I can do this!

☐ Committed—I will follow
   through even if I falter here
   and there

☐ Defeated—need to
   remind myself that every
   little bit counts

Took time for myself   [Yes] [No]

Relaxed   [Yes] [No]

accomplishments!

_____
_____
_____
_____
_____
_____
_____
_____
_____

☐ Weight loss? _____
☐ Waist measurement: _____
☐ Blood sugar improvement?

_____
_____

"We never repent
of having eaten too
little."
—Thomas Jefferson

next week's goals

eat Focus on eating more
often—the best way to keep your
blood sugar steady and rev your
metabolism so you burn more
calories. Aim for three balanced
meals and two snacks of about
150 calories each.

move You should have started the DMS walking plan by
now. Next week, work on setting
your new habit in stone. Put
your walks on your calendar, and
be sure to keep all your
"appointments."

choose Enlist a support
team. Ask your spouse to join
you in your walks next week.
Tell all your friends and family
that you've started to improve
your diet, and solicit their
encouragement.

10 super foods for better diabetes control

Eating right is key to managing diabetes. Fortunately, your food "prescription" includes filling, flavorful fare that tastes like anything but medicine. A diet rich in these 10 "super-foods" will help minimize blood sugar swings, provide key nutrients (such as magnesium, which many people with diabetes need more of), and help you step lighter on the scale—a proven way to lower your blood sugar and even throw your disease into reverse. Dig in!

*1 vegetables

The advantages of eating more vegetables are undeniable. Packed with powerhouse nutrients, vegetables are naturally low in calories, and they're full of fiber, so they're plenty filling. Loading your plate with more vegetables will automatically mean you're eating fewer simple carbs (which raise blood sugar) and saturated fats (which increase insulin resistance). Aim to get four or five servings a day. (A serving is 1/2 cup canned or cooked vegetables or 1 cup raw vegetables.) Go easier on starchy vegetables—including potatoes and corn, and legumes such as lima beans and peas—which are higher in calories than other vegetables.

*2 beans

Beans are just about your best source of dietary fiber. Fiber slows digestion and keeps blood sugar from rising quickly after a meal. This effect is so powerful that it can even lower your overall blood sugar levels. Because it slows digestion, fiber also keeps you feeling full longer.

Throw canned beans into every salad you make (rinse them first), and add them to pasta dishes and chili. Black bean, split pea, or lentil soup, even it comes from a can, is an excellent lunch.

*3 fruit

It has more natural sugar and calories than most vegetables, so you can't eat it with utter abandon, but fruit has almost all the advantages that vegetables do—it's brimming with nutrients you need, it's low in fat, it's high in fiber, and it's relatively low in calories compared with most other foods. Best of all, it's loaded with antioxidants that help protect your nerves, your eyes, and your heart.

Aim to get three or four servings a day. (A serving is one piece of whole fruit, 1/2 cup cooked or canned fruit, or 1 cup raw fruit.) Strive to make most of your fruit servings real produce, not juice. Many of the nutrients and a lot of the fiber found in the skin, flesh, and seeds of fruit are eliminated during juicing, and the calories and sugar are concentrated in juice.

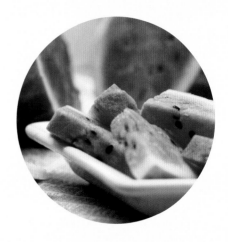

*4 yogurt

Yogurt is rich in protein and something else important for weight loss: calcium. Several studies have shown that people who eat plenty of calcium-rich foods have an easier time losing weight—and are less likely to become insulin resistant. As a snack or for breakfast, choose nonfat plain yogurt, and add your own fresh fruit or a sprinkling of wheat germ or low-fat granola for a burst of extra nutrients.

*5 cereal

The right breakfast cereal is your absolute best opportunity to pack more fiber into your day. There's a bonus: Studies show that people who start the morning with a high-fiber cereal actually eat less later on. So don't forgo breakfast. And choose a cereal brand with at least 5 grams fiber per serving. Good choices include Kashi GoLean Crunch! (10 grams), Kellogg's Raisin Bran (8 grams), General Mills Multi-Bran Chex (8 grams), Post Wheat 'N Bran Spoon Size (8 grams), Kellogg's All-Bran Original (10 grams) and General Mills Fiber One (14 grams). Top your cereal with fruit and you've checked off a fruit serving for the day.

*6 fish

Fast and easy to prepare, fish is a good source of protein, and a great substitute for higher-fat meats. Fatty fish is also the best source of omega-3 fatty acids, those remarkable good-for-you fats that help keep the arteries clear. People with diabetes often have high triglycerides and low levels of HDL, the "good" cholesterol. Omega-3 fatty acids can improve both numbers. Aim to eat fish at least twice a week. Excellent sources of omega-3s are salmon, mackerel, and tuna.

*7 chicken breast

Versatile, extremely lean, and low in calories, chicken breast is practically a miracle food. Unlike steaks and hamburgers, it's low in saturated fat, which raises "bad" cholesterol and may increase insulin resistance, making blood sugar control more difficult. A 3-ounce serving of skinless chicken breast has only 142 calories and 3 grams fat. Turkey breast is even leaner and lower in calories.

*8 nuts

Nuts have several things going for them—and for you. They're loaded with "good" fats that fight heart disease. These fats have even been shown to help reduce insulin resistance and make blood sugar easier to control. Nuts are also one of the best food sources of vitamin E, an antioxidant that protects cells and may help prevent nerve and eye damage. They are rich in fiber and magnesium, both of which may benefit your blood sugar. Studies suggest that including them in your diet may even help you lose weight. Because nuts are high in calories, though, eat them in moderation.

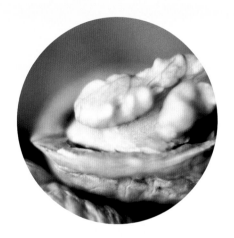

*9 olive oil ✗

At the dead center of the famously heart-healthy Mediterranean diet is olive oil, full of "good" fats that slash the risk of heart attack—and help keep blood sugar steady. These fats have even been shown to help reduce insulin resistance. So toss the butter and cook with olive oil instead. At home and in restaurants, dip your bread in a bit of the stuff. Just watch how much you eat, because at 9 calories per gram, even the "good" fat in olive oil can pack on the pounds.

*10 cinnamon ✗

Believe it! Amazingly, just by sprinkling cinnamon on your foods, you could lower your blood sugar. Components in cinnamon help the body use insulin more efficiently, so more glucose can enter cells. A recent study found that in people with diabetes, just 1/2 teaspoon a day can significantly lower blood sugar levels. So go ahead and add powdered cinnamon to your whole wheat toast, oatmeal, baked apples, or even chicken dishes. Or soak a cinnamon stick in hot water to make a soothing and curative cup of cinnamon tea.

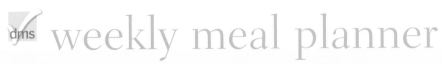

weekly meal planner

date   **Monday**   **Tuesday**   **Wednesday**

On the DMS, we want you to eat five times a day: three moderate-sized meals, plus two healthy snacks. That means you should never skip breakfast.

What's a healthy breakfast for people with diabetes? One that's high in fiber and also contains some protein. Good choices that fit the bill:

• A bowl of high-fiber cereal topped with fresh fruit

• A cup of low-fat yogurt with fresh fruit and a cereal bar

• A vegetable omelet with one slice whole wheat toast

• A mini whole wheat bagel with 2 table-spoons peanut butter

• A bowl of oatmeal topped with cinnamon and walnuts

breakfast

lunch

dinner

Thursday   Friday   Saturday   Sunday

Food Fact Sweet potatoes are higher in fiber and nutrients
and have less impact on blood sugar than white potatoes.

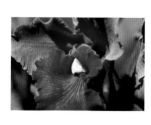

dms

monday

my numbers

weight _____   blood sugar (time/level) _____ / _____ ● _____ / _____ ● _____ / _____ ● _____ / _____

what I ate today

circle the number of servings

fruit

0 1 2 3 **4**

vegetables

0 1 2 3 4 **5**

whole grains

0 1 2 3 4 5 **6**

calcium-rich foods

0 1 **2** 3

beans

0 1 2

fish

0 1 2

extra lean poultry or meat

0 1 2

glasses of water

0 1 2 3 4 5 6 **7 8** 9 10

times I ate out of boredom, stress, or habit

0 1 2 3 4 5

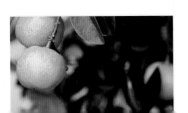

✴ **Tip of the day** - Treat exercise like a doctor's appointment. Decide when you're going to do it, and write it down in your date book in ink. Take it as seriously as any other important appointment. You wouldn't skip a visit to the doctor just because you didn't feel like going; you shouldn't miss a workout for that reason either.

taking charge of my health!

eat

☐ ate a healthy breakfast
☐ had protein at every meal
☐ had 1-2 healthy snacks
☐ ate dinner by 7:00 p.m.
☐ avoided "white" foods
☐ drank water or tea instead of sugary drinks

move

☐ walked _____ steps/minutes
☐ made active choices
☐ got other exercise

_____

choose

☐ took my vitamins
☐ got enough sleep _____ hrs
☐ kept TV time under 2 hours

successes & confessions

rate your attitude today

3 excellent
2 good
1 so-so
0 disaster! plan to do better tomorrow

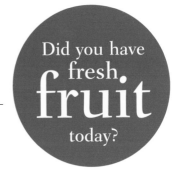

Did you have fresh. **fruit** today?

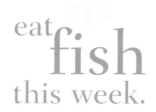

tuesday

my numbers

weight _____   blood sugar (time/level) _____ / _____ • _____ / _____ • _____ / _____ • _____ / _____

✳ **Tip of the day** - Share the news. Tell family and friends that you are starting an exercise/weight-loss program and that you would like their support. Who knows—they may join you in your efforts to eat better. Perhaps they'd even like to be your exercise buddy.

taking charge of my health!

eat

☐ ate a healthy breakfast
☐ had protein at every meal
☐ had 1-2 healthy snacks
☐ ate dinner by 7:00 p.m.
☐ avoided "white" foods
☐ drank water or tea instead of sugary drinks

move

☐ walked _____ steps/minutes
☐ made active choices
☐ got other exercise

_____

choose

☐ took my vitamins
☐ got enough sleep _____ hrs
☐ kept TV time under 2 hours

successes & confessions

rate your attitude today

3   excellent
2   good
1   so-so
0   disaster! plan to do better tomorrow

what I ate today

circle the number of servings

fruit

0 1 2 3 **4**

vegetables

0 1 2 3 4 **5**

whole grains

0 1 2 3 4 5 **6**

calcium-rich foods

0 1 **2** **3**

beans

0 1 2

fish

0 1 2

extra lean poultry or meat

0 1 2

glasses of water

0 1 2 3 4 5 6 **7** **8** 9 10

times I ate out of boredom, stress, or habit

0 **1** 2 3 4 5

eat. **fish** this week.

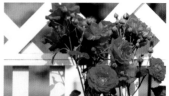

dms

wednesday

my numbers

weight _____   blood sugar (time/level) _____ / _____ • _____ / _____ • _____ / _____ • _____ / _____

what I ate today

circle the number of servings

fruit

0 1 2 3 **4**

vegetables

0 1 2 3 4 **5**

whole grains

0 1 2 3 4 5 **6**

calcium-rich foods

0 1 **2** 3

beans

0 1 2

fish

0 1 2

extra lean poultry or meat

0 1 2

glasses of water

0 1 2 3 4 5 6 **7** **8** 9 10

times I ate out of boredom, stress, or habit

0 **1** 2 3 4 5

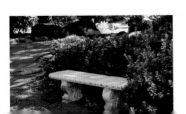

✳ Tip of the day - Be sure to keep track of your walking or other exercise every day. Filling in those spaces on these pages helps you stay true to your commitment and gives you a great sense of satisfaction—how exciting to look back and see that you've met your weekly exercise goals three weeks in a row, and that you've lost three pounds!

taking charge of my health!

eat

☐ ate a healthy breakfast
☐ had protein at every meal
☐ had 1-2 healthy snacks
☐ ate dinner by 7:00 p.m.
☐ avoided "white" foods
☐ drank water or tea instead of sugary drinks

move

☐ walked _____ steps/minutes
☐ made active choices
☐ got other exercise

_____

choose

☐ took my vitamins
☐ got enough sleep _____ hrs
☐ kept TV time under 2 hours

successes & confessions

rate your attitude today

3 excellent
2 good
1 so-so
0 disaster! plan to do better tomorrow

Did you go somewhere **green** today?

thursday

my numbers

weight _____ blood sugar (time/level) _____ / _____ ● _____ / _____ ● _____ / _____ ● _____ / _____

✳ **Tip of the day** - For recipes that call for the smoky taste of bacon (soups, chowders, egg dishes, and bean dishes), choose lean turkey bacon instead of pork bacon. It delivers plenty of flavor while saving significantly on calories and fat. Experiment to find a brand you like.

what I ate today

circle the number of servings

fruit

0 1 2 3 **4**

vegetables

0 1 2 3 4 **5**

whole grains

0 1 2 3 4 5 **6**

calcium-rich foods

0 1 **2** 3

beans

0 1 2

fish

0 1 2

extra lean poultry or meat

0 1 2

glasses of water

0 1 2 3 4 5 6 **7 8** 9 10

times I ate out of boredom, stress, or habit

0 1 2 3 4 5

taking charge of my health!

eat
- ☐ ate a healthy breakfast
- ☐ had protein at every meal
- ☐ had 1-2 healthy snacks
- ☐ ate dinner by 7:00 p.m.
- ☐ avoided "white" foods
- ☐ drank water or tea instead of sugary drinks

move
- ☐ walked _____ steps/minutes
- ☐ made active choices
- ☐ got other exercise
- ☐ _____

choose
- ☐ took my vitamins
- ☐ got enough sleep _____ hrs
- ☐ kept TV time under 2 hours

successes & confessions

rate your attitude today

3 excellent
2 good
1 so-so
0 disaster! plan to do better tomorrow

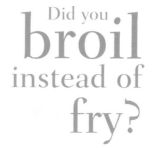

Did you **broil** instead of **fry?**

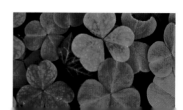

my numbers

weight _____   blood sugar (time/level) _____ / _____ • _____ / _____ • _____ / _____ • _____ / _____

what I ate today

circle the number of servings

fruit

0 1 2 3 **4**

vegetables

0 1 2 3 4 **5**

whole grains

0 1 2 3 4 5 **6**

calcium-rich foods

0 1 **2** 3

beans

0 1 2

fish

0 1 2

extra lean poultry or meat

0 1 2

glasses of water

0 1 2 3 4 5 6 **7** **8** 9 10

times I ate out of boredom, stress, or habit

0 **1** 2 3 4 5

※ Tip of the day - Don't wear worn-out sneakers. If you walk or run, your sneakers will carry you about 350 to 500 miles; after that, the cushioning is so compressed that your feet won't be adequately supported. If you're walking 15 miles a week, that means replacing your sneakers every six months.

taking charge of my health!

eat

☐ ate a healthy breakfast
☐ had protein at every meal
☐ had 1-2 healthy snacks
☐ ate dinner by 7:00 p.m.
☐ avoided "white" foods
☐ drank water or tea instead of sugary drinks

move

☐ walked _____ steps/minutes
☐ made active choices
☐ got other exercise
_____

choose

☐ took my vitamins
☐ got enough sleep _____ hrs
☐ kept TV time under 2 hours

rate your attitude today

3 excellent
2 good
1 so-so
0 disaster! plan to do better tomorrow

Start your day with a positive attitude.

successes & confessions

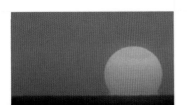

saturday

dms

my numbers

weight _____   blood sugar (time/level) _____ / _____ • _____ / _____ • _____ / _____ • _____ / _____

❋ **Tip of the day** - Choose whole wheat pasta. It's denser than regular white pasta, with a firm texture similar to what you'd get in Italy. Top it with a high-fiber sauce, such as mixed vegetables (pasta primavera) or beans (pasta e fagioli). The fiber in the toppings will help limit the rise in blood sugar caused by the pasta.

taking charge of my health!

eat
- ☐ ate a healthy breakfast
- ☐ had protein at every meal
- ☐ had 1-2 healthy snacks
- ☐ ate dinner by 7:00 p.m.
- ☐ avoided "white" foods
- ☐ drank water or tea instead of sugary drinks

move
- ☐ walked _____ steps/minutes
- ☐ made active choices
- ☐ got other exercise
- _____

choose
- ☐ took my vitamins
- ☐ got enough sleep _____ hrs
- ☐ kept TV time under 2 hours

successes & confessions

rate your attitude today
3 excellent
2 good
1 so-so
0 disaster! plan to do better tomorrow

Reward yourself for a recent success.

what I ate today

circle the number of servings

fruit
0 1 2 3 **4**

vegetables
0 1 2 3 4 **5**

whole grains
0 1 2 3 4 5 **6**

calcium-rich foods
0 1 **2** 3

beans
0 1 2

fish
0 1 2

extra lean poultry or meat
0 1 2

glasses of water
0 1 2 3 4 5 6 **7** **8** 9 10

times I ate out of boredom, stress, or habit
0 **1** 2 3 4 5

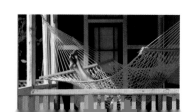

sunday

my numbers

weight _____   blood sugar (time/level) _____ / _____ ◦ _____ / _____ ◦ _____ / _____ ◦ _____ / _____

what I ate today

circle the number of servings

fruit

0 1 2 3 **4**

vegetables

0 1 2 3 4 **5**

whole grains

0 1 2 3 4 5 **6**

calcium-rich foods

0 1 **2** **3**

beans

0 1 2

fish

0 1 2

extra lean poultry or meat

0 1 2

glasses of water

0 1 2 3 4 5 6 **7** **8** 9 10

times I ate out of boredom, stress, or habit

0 **1** 2 3 4 5

✳ Tip of the day - Exercise can cause blood sugar levels to rise or fall, so it's important to monitor your blood sugar before and after exercising. If your blood sugar is less than 100 mg/dl, have a snack, such as a piece of fruit, before you exercise. Don't exercise if your blood sugar level is less than 100 mg/dl.

taking charge of my health!

eat

☐ ate a healthy breakfast
☐ had protein at every meal
☐ had 1-2 healthy snacks
☐ ate dinner by 7:00 p.m.
☐ avoided "white" foods
☐ drank water or tea instead of sugary drinks

move

☐ walked _____ steps/minutes
☐ made active choices
☐ got other exercise

_____

choose

☐ took my vitamins
☐ got enough sleep _____ hrs
☐ kept TV time under 2 hours

rate your attitude today

3 excellent
2 good
1 so-so
0 disaster! plan to do better
    tomorrow

Have you
checked your
feet
for injuries?

successes & confessions

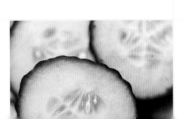

week in review & ahead >

how well I did

eat

Improved my eating
from previous week   *[Yes] [No]*

Made healthy
restaurant choices   *[Yes] [No]*

Tried a new fruit,
vegetable, or grain   *[Yes] [No]*

move

Total walking time _____

Total steps _____
(if using a pedometer)

Walked more than
I did previous week   *[Yes] [No]*

Moved more than
I did previous week   *[Yes] [No]*

Felt more energized
than previous week   *[Yes] [No]*

choose

My attitude this week was:

☐ Positive—I can do this!

☐ Committed—I will follow
   through even if I falter here
   and there

☐ Defeated—need to
   remind myself that every
   little bit counts

Took time for myself   *[Yes] [No]*

Relaxed   *[Yes] [No]*

accomplishments!

_____
_____
_____
_____
_____
_____
_____
_____
_____

☐ Weight loss? _____
☐ Waist measurement: _____
☐ Blood sugar improvement?

_____
_____

> " To eat
> is a necessity, but to
> eat intelligently
> is an art. "
>
> —La Rochefoucauld

next week's goals

eat Eat breakfast every day
next week, and make it a good
one. Stock up on cereals that contain 5 grams of fiber per serving,
and top them with fresh fruit.

move Increase your walking
time. Your goal next week: 20
minutes of walking on five days.
Any pace is fine for now.

choose Getting a good
night's sleep is critical to helping
you stay the course. If you're
not getting a full 8 hours (or
however many hours you need
to feel truly rested), move up
your bedtime by an hour.

15 ways to cut
50 calories
or more

Think small! Trimming even just a small percentage of your body weight can do wonders for your blood sugar. And eating just a bit less is the way to do it. Shaving calories here and there is easier than you think. All it takes are a few no-sweat efforts like the ones that follow. Pick two a day and you'll cut 100 calories. Burn 100 more calories a day (a 15- to 20-minute walk will do the trick) and you'll lose almost half a pound a week. That may not sound like much, but it adds up to 20 pounds a year!

1. Leave the cheese off your sandwich. 2. Use 1 cup skim milk instead of 1 cup whole milk. 3. Substitute 4 ounces ground turkey for 4 ounces ground beef. 4. Eat 2 tablespoons less ice cream. 5. Order small fries instead of large fries. 6. Substitute 1 tablespoon jam for 1 tablespoon butter. 7. Use 1 tablespoon light mayonnaise instead of 1 tablespoon regular mayo. 8. Use one less pat of margarine 9. Have 1 ounce of pretzels instead of 1 ounce of potato chips. 10. Use 1 tablespoon less salad dressing. 11. Have an English muffin instead of a doughnut 12. Use 1 tablespoon less cream cheese. 13. Drink 4 ounces less juice. 14. Use a non-stick spray instead of 2 teaspoons oil 15. Drink seltzer or diet soda instead of regular soda.

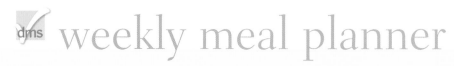

weekly meal planner

date	Monday	Tuesday	Wednesday
breakfast			
lunch			
dinner			

Plan at least one vegetarian meal this week. Try Chili with White Beans, Tomatoes, and Corn (recipe card attached). Need more recipe ideas? The Moosewood Restaurant cookbook series is popular, and for good reason. Other good options: *Cooking Vegetarian: Healthy, Delicious, and Easy Vegetarian Cuisine*, and *Becoming Vegetarian: The Complete Guide to Adopting a Healthy Vegetarian Diet*.

To get more vegetables into your meals, take advantage of prepared veggies—bagged salads, prewashed spinach, chopped bell peppers and onions, etc. Also, stock the freezer with bags of frozen vegetables and use them in stir-fries.

Thursday   Friday   Saturday   Sunday

Food Fact One tablespoon of ketchup contains about half a
teaspoon of sugar. Buying sugar-free condiments can
make a dent in your overall sugar consumption.

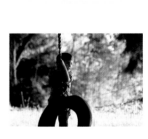

monday

my numbers

weight _____ blood sugar (time/level) _____ / _____ • _____ / _____ • _____ / _____ • _____ / _____

what I ate today

circle the number of servings

fruit

0 1 2 3 **4**

vegetables

0 1 2 3 4 **5**

whole grains

0 1 2 3 4 5 **6**

calcium-rich foods

0 1 **2** **3**

beans

0 1 2

fish

0 1 2

extra lean poultry or meat

0 1 2

glasses of water

0 1 2 3 4 5 6 **7** **8** 9 10

times I ate out of boredom, stress, or habit

0 **1** 2 3 4 5

❋ **Tip of the day** - Skew your diet to fresh foods instead of processed foods. If you make vegetables, fruits, whole grains, fish, poultry, and lean meat the mainstays of your diet and avoid processed foods, including cakes, chips, candy, and just about anything that comes out of a box (except rice or pasta), you'll be much more likely to lose weight.

taking charge of my health!

eat

☐ ate a healthy breakfast

☐ had protein at every meal

☐ had 1-2 healthy snacks

☐ ate dinner by 7:00 p.m.

☐ avoided "white" foods

☐ drank water or tea instead of sugary drinks

move

☐ walked _____ steps/minutes

☐ made active choices

☐ got other exercise

_____

choose

☐ took my vitamins

☐ got enough sleep _____ hrs

☐ kept TV time under 2 hours

successes & confessions

rate your attitude today

3 excellent

2 good

1 so-so

0 disaster! plan to do better tomorrow

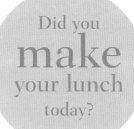

Did you **make** your lunch today?

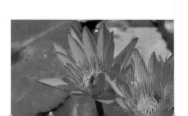

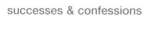

tuesday

my numbers

weight _____ blood sugar (time/level) _____ / _____ • _____ / _____ • _____ / _____ • _____ / _____

✳ **Tip of the day** - Don't push too hard. When you exercise, check the intensity of your workout. Are you gasping for breath? Is your heart beating wildly? Do you feel completely worn out by the end? If so, lighten up. Moderate-intensity exercise is effective, and it's easier to adhere to. When you work out too hard, it feels like punishment, and you won't want to do it again the next day.

taking charge of my health!

eat
- ☐ ate a healthy breakfast
- ☐ had protein at every meal
- ☐ had 1-2 healthy snacks
- ☐ ate dinner by 7:00 p.m.
- ☐ avoided "white" foods
- ☐ drank water or tea instead of sugary drinks

move
- ☐ walked _____ steps/minutes
- ☐ made active choices
- ☐ got other exercise
- _____

choose
- ☐ took my vitamins
- ☐ got enough sleep _____ hrs
- ☐ kept TV time under 2 hours

successes & confessions

rate your attitude today
3   excellent
2   good
1   so-so
0   disaster! plan to do better tomorrow

what I ate today

circle the number of servings

fruit
0 1 2 3 **4**

vegetables
0 1 2 3 4 **5**

whole grains
0 1 2 3 4 5 **6**

calcium-rich foods
0 1 **2** **3**

beans
0 1 2

fish
0 1 2

extra lean poultry or meat
0 1 2

glasses of water
0 1 2 3 4 5 6 **7** **8** 9 10

times I ate out of boredom, stress, or habit
0 **1** 2 3 4 5

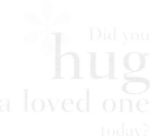

Did you *hug* a loved one today?

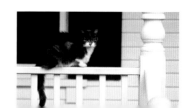

wednesday

my numbers

weight _____   blood sugar (time/level) _____ / _____ • _____ / _____ • _____ / _____ • _____ / _____

what I ate today

circle the number of servings

fruit

0 1 2 3 **4**

vegetables

0 1 2 3 4 **5**

whole grains

0 1 2 3 4 5 **6**

calcium-rich foods

0 1 **2** **3**

beans

0 1 2

fish

0 1 2

extra lean poultry or meat

0 1 2

glasses of water

0 1 2 3 4 5 6 **7** **8** 9 10

times I ate out of boredom, stress, or habit

0 **1** 2 3 4 5

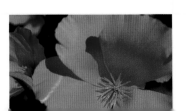

✳ **Tip of the day** - Never let yourself get too hungry. If you're starving, you're more likely to eat whatever's available—and you'll probably eat too much. Keep packets of peanuts, small cartons of fat-free yogurt, carrot slices, cans of vegetable juice, and other healthy snacks at home, in the car, or in the office, and have a snack midway between meals.

taking charge of my health!

eat

☐ ate a healthy breakfast

☐ had protein at every meal

☐ had 1-2 healthy snacks

☐ ate dinner by 7:00 p.m.

☐ avoided "white" foods

☐ drank water or tea instead of sugary drinks

move

☐ walked _____ steps/minutes

☐ made active choices

☐ got other exercise

_____

choose

☐ took my vitamins

☐ got enough sleep _____ hrs

☐ kept TV time under 2 hours

successes & confessions

rate your attitude today

3 excellent

2 good

1 so-so

0 disaster! plan to do better tomorrow

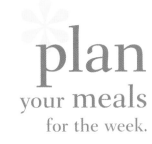

✳ plan

your meals

for the week.

thursday

my numbers

weight _____ blood sugar (time/level) _____ / _____ ⚹ _____ / _____ ⚹ _____ / _____ ⚹ _____ / _____

✳ **Tip of the day** - Beans are an excellent food for weight loss and nutrition. Add canned black, white, or red beans (rinse them first) to salads and pasta to bulk up your meal. Just watch out for the refried kind: Many are mixed with lard, which is high in calories, saturated fat, and cholesterol. If you buy refried beans, look for a fat-free brand.

taking charge of my health!

eat
☐ ate a healthy breakfast
☐ had protein at every meal
☐ had 1-2 healthy snacks
☐ ate dinner by 7:00 p.m.
☐ avoided "white" foods
☐ drank water or tea instead of sugary drinks

move
☐ walked _____ steps/minutes
☐ made active choices
☐ got other exercise
_____

choose
☐ took my vitamins
☐ got enough sleep _____ hrs
☐ kept TV time under 2 hours

successes & confessions

rate your attitude today
3 excellent
2 good
1 so-so
0 disaster! plan to do better tomorrow

Catch up with a
friend
who makes you
feel good.

what I ate today

circle the number of servings

fruit
0 1 2 3 **4**

vegetables
0 1 2 3 4 **5**

whole grains
0 1 2 3 4 5 **6**

calcium-rich foods
0 1 **2** **3**

beans
0 1 2

fish
0 1 2

extra lean poultry or meat
0 1 2

glasses of water
0 1 2 3 4 5 6 **7** **8** 9 10

times I ate out of boredom, stress, or habit
0 **1** 2 3 4 5

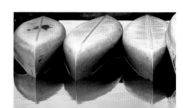

friday

my numbers

weight _____   blood sugar (time/level) _____ / _____ ∗ _____ / _____ ∗ _____ / _____ ∗ _____ / _____

what I ate today

circle the number of servings

fruit

0 1 2 3 **4**

vegetables

0 1 2 3 4 **5**

whole grains

0 1 2 3 4 5 **6**

calcium-rich foods

0 1 **2** **3**

beans

0 1 2

fish

0 1 2

extra lean poultry or meat

0 1 2

glasses of water

0 1 2 3 4 5 6 **7** **8** 9 10

times I ate out of boredom, stress, or habit

0 **1** 2 3 4 5

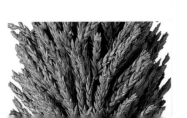

✳ Tip of the day - In recipes that call for whole eggs, save calories, saturated fat, and cholesterol by substituting egg whites instead. Replace each egg in the recipe with two egg whites. Or use a cholesterol-free liquid egg product instead. When buying eggs, consider a brand enriched with omega-3 fatty acids, which benefit your heart health.

taking charge of my health!

eat

☐ ate a healthy breakfast

☐ had protein at every meal

☐ had 1-2 healthy snacks

☐ ate dinner by 7:00 p.m.

☐ avoided "white" foods

☐ drank water or tea instead of sugary drinks

move

☐ walked _____ steps/minutes

☐ made active choices

☐ got other exercise

_____

choose

☐ took my vitamins

☐ got enough sleep _____ hrs

☐ kept TV time under 2 hours

successes & confessions

rate your attitude today

3 excellent

2 good

1 so-so

0 disaster! plan to do better tomorrow

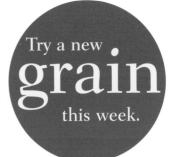

Try a new **grain** this week.

saturday

my numbers

weight _____ blood sugar (time/level) _____ / _____ • _____ / _____ • _____ / _____ • _____ / _____

❊ **Tip of the day** - Watch your posture when you walk. Hold your body fully upright, with your shoulders pulled slightly back and down. Keep your arms bent at a 90-degree angle. Don't thrust your head forward. Instead, keep your ears aligned with your shoulders. Your hands should be lightly clenched.

taking charge of my health!

eat

- ☐ ate a healthy breakfast
- ☐ had protein at every meal
- ☐ had 1-2 healthy snacks
- ☐ ate dinner by 7:00 p.m.
- ☐ avoided "white" foods
- ☐ drank water or tea instead of sugary drinks

move

- ☐ walked _____ steps/minutes
- ☐ made active choices
- ☐ got other exercise
- _____

choose

- ☐ took my vitamins
- ☐ got enough sleep _____ hrs
- ☐ kept TV time under 2 hours

successes & confessions

rate your attitude today

3   excellent
2   good
1   so-so
0   disaster! plan to do better tomorrow

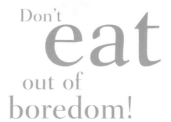

Don't **eat** out of boredom!

what I ate today

circle the number of servings

fruit

0 1 2 3 **4**

vegetables

0 1 2 3 4 **5**

whole grains

0 1 2 3 4 5 **6**

calcium-rich foods

0 1 **2** **3**

beans

0 1 2

fish

0 1 2

extra lean poultry or meat

0 1 2

glasses of water

0 1 2 3 4 5 6 **7** **8** 9 10

times I ate out of boredom, stress, or habit

0 **1** 2 3 4 5

sunday

my numbers

weight _____ blood sugar (time/level) _____ / _____ • _____ / _____ • _____ / _____ • _____ / _____

what I ate today

circle the number of servings

fruit

0 1 2 3 **4**

vegetables

0 1 2 3 4 **5**

whole grains

0 1 2 3 4 5 **6**

calcium-rich foods

0 1 **2 3**

beans

0 1 2

fish

0 1 2

extra lean poultry or meat

0 1 2

glasses of water

0 1 2 3 4 5 6 **7 8** 9 10

times I ate out of boredom, stress, or habit

0 1 2 3 4 5

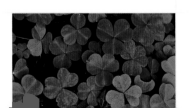

✳ **Tip of the day** - If you find yourself in a situation in which there's nothing to eat but fast food, make smart choices that will be good for your blood sugar and your waistline. Order a salad with low-cal dressing, if it's on the menu. If not, a small ("junior") hamburger, a small order of fries, and a diet soda add up to only 477 calories. A grilled chicken sandwich (no mayo) is another good choice.

taking charge of my health!

eat

☐ ate a healthy breakfast
☐ had protein at every meal
☐ had 1-2 healthy snacks
☐ ate dinner by 7:00 p.m.
☐ avoided "white" foods
☐ drank water or tea instead of sugary drinks

rate your attitude today

3 excellent
2 good
1 so-so
0 disaster! plan to do better tomorrow

move

☐ walked _____ steps/minutes
☐ made active choices
☐ got other exercise

_____

choose

☐ took my vitamins
☐ got enough sleep _____ hrs
☐ kept TV time under 2 hours

successes & confessions

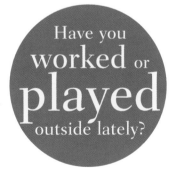

Have you **worked** or **played** outside lately?

week in review & ahead >

how well I did

eat

Improved my eating
from previous week   *[Yes] [No]*

Made healthy
restaurant choices   *[Yes] [No]*

Tried a new fruit,
vegetable, or grain   *[Yes] [No]*

move

Total walking time _____

Total steps _____
(if using a pedometer)

Walked more than
I did previous week   *[Yes] [No]*

Moved more than
I did previous week   *[Yes] [No]*

Felt more energized
than previous week   *[Yes] [No]*

choose

My attitude this week was:

☐ Positive—I can do this!

☐ Committed—I will follow
through even if I falter here
and there

☐ Defeated—need to
remind myself that every
little bit counts

Took time for myself   *[Yes] [No]*

Relaxed   *[Yes] [No]*

accomplishments!

_____
_____
_____
_____
_____
_____
_____
_____
_____

☐ Weight loss? _____
☐ Waist measurement: _____
☐ Blood sugar improvement?

_____
_____

*❝It is not work that
kills men; it is worry.
… Fear secretes acids;
but love and trust are
sweet juices.❞*

—Henry Ward Beecher

next week's goals

eat Focus on eating more vegetables. Start lunch and dinner with a salad, and add color (in the form of veggies) to every meal you make.

move Improve your walking posture. Stand tall with your spine elongated and breastbone lifted. Avoid slumping your shoulders forward or hunching them toward your ears. Pull in your tummy.

choose Practice deep breathing for 5 minutes every day next week. Breathe deeply through your nose, expanding your belly and filling your lungs from the bottom up. Exhale slowly.

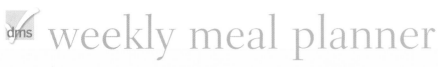

weekly meal planner

date	Monday	Tuesday	Wednesday

Cook up a whole grain to go with dinner. Try pearl barley (which doesn't require any soaking before cooking) as a side dish. Or mix in some steamed carrots and broccoli, toss with olive oil and a bit of Parmesan or feta cheese, maybe throw in a can of tuna or a couple of ounces of cut-up chicken, and you've got the whole dinner.

`For a delicious high-fiber meal, make Barley Risotto with Asparagus and Mushrooms (recipe card attached). Other interesting grains to experiment with include amaranth and wheat berries.

breakfast

lunch

dinner

	Thursday	Friday	Saturday	Sunday

Food Fact One-half cup of vanilla frozen yogurt has just 100 calories compared with 160 calories or more for one-half cup of premium ice cream.

monday

my numbers

weight _____ blood sugar (time/level) _____ / _____ • _____ / _____ • _____ / _____ • _____ / _____

what I ate today

circle the number of servings

fruit

0 1 2 3 **4**

vegetables

0 1 2 3 4 **5**

whole grains

0 1 2 3 4 5 **6**

calcium-rich foods

0 1 **2** **3**

beans

0 1 2

fish

0 1 2

extra lean poultry or meat

0 1 2

glasses of water

0 1 2 3 4 5 6 **7** **8** 9 10

times I ate out of boredom, stress, or habit

0 **1** 2 3 4 5

※ **Tip of the day** - Buy a pedometer. These little gadgets keep track of all of your steps during the day—not only when you're walking for exercise, but when you're going down the hall to talk to your boss, striding to the train or bus, or chasing after a toddler. Pedometers are available at sporting-goods stores. Aim for a goal of 10,000 steps a day.

taking charge of my health!

eat

☐ ate a healthy breakfast

☐ had protein at every meal

☐ had 1-2 healthy snacks

☐ ate dinner by 7:00 p.m.

☐ avoided "white" foods

☐ drank water or tea instead of sugary drinks

move

☐ walked _____ steps/minutes

☐ made active choices

☐ got other exercise

_____

choose

☐ took my vitamins

☐ got enough sleep _____ hrs

☐ kept TV time under 2 hours

successes & confessions

rate your attitude today

3 excellent

2 good

1 so-so

0 disaster! plan to do better tomorrow

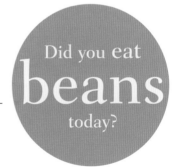

Did you eat **beans** today?

dms

tuesday

my numbers

weight _____ blood sugar (time/level) _____ / _____ • _____ / _____ • _____ / _____ • _____ / _____

* Tip of the day - Eat "wet" foods. Studies show that foods that contain liquid—grapes, soups, stews, and smoothies, for example—make you feel fuller than a dry food with the same number of calories. A 100-calorie bowl of soup will leave you feeling fuller than a 100-calorie bag of pretzels. An exception: soda. The empty calories in soda don't seem to trigger fullness.

taking charge of my health!

eat

- ☐ ate a healthy breakfast
- ☐ had protein at every meal
- ☐ had 1-2 healthy snacks
- ☐ ate dinner by 7:00 p.m.
- ☐ avoided "white" foods
- ☐ drank water or tea instead of sugary drinks

move

- ☐ walked _____ steps/minutes
- ☐ made active choices
- ☐ got other exercise
- _____

choose

- ☐ took my vitamins
- ☐ got enough sleep _____ hrs
- ☐ kept TV time under 2 hours

successes & confessions

rate your attitude today

3 excellent
2 good
1 so-so
0 disaster! plan to do better tomorrow

what I ate today

circle the number of servings

fruit

0 1 2 3 **4**

vegetables

0 1 2 3 4 **5**

whole grains

0 1 2 3 4 5 **6**

calcium-rich foods

0 1 **2** 3

beans

0 1 2

fish

0 1 2

extra lean poultry or meat

0 1 2

glasses of water

0 1 2 3 4 5 6 **7** **8** 9 10

times I ate out of boredom, stress, or habit

0 **1** 2 3 4 5

Go to
sleep
on time tonight!

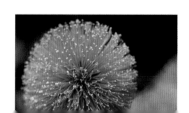

wednesday

my numbers

weight _____ blood sugar (time/level) _____ / _____ • _____ / _____ • _____ / _____ • _____ / _____

what I ate today

circle the number of servings

fruit

0 1 2 3 **4**

vegetables

0 1 2 3 4 **5**

whole grains

0 1 2 3 4 5 **6**

calcium-rich foods

0 1 **2** 3

beans

0 1 2

fish

0 1 2

extra lean poultry or meat

0 1 2

glasses of water

0 1 2 3 4 5 6 **7** **8** 9 10

times I ate out of boredom, stress, or habit

0 **1** 2 3 4 5

* Tip of the day - Hunger isn't the only reason we reach for food. Boredom, anger, sadness, and stress sometimes inspire an eating spree even when we're not really hungry. The next time you find yourself reaching for a chocolate bar, think about why you want it. Maybe taking a bath, writing in a journal, calling a friend, or taking a walk will make you feel better instead.

taking charge of my health!

eat

☐ ate a healthy breakfast
☐ had protein at every meal
☐ had 1-2 healthy snacks
☐ ate dinner by 7:00 p.m.
☐ avoided "white" foods
☐ drank water or tea instead of sugary drinks

move

☐ walked _____ steps/minutes
☐ made active choices
☐ got other exercise

_____

choose

☐ took my vitamins
☐ got enough sleep _____ hrs
☐ kept TV time under 2 hours

rate your attitude today

3 excellent
2 good
1 so-so
0 disaster! plan to do better tomorrow

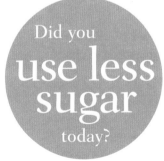

Did you **use less sugar** today?

successes & confessions

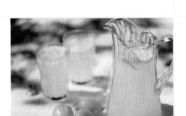

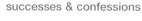

thursday

my numbers

weight _____   blood sugar (time/level) _____ / _____ • _____ / _____ • _____ / _____ • _____ / _____

☀ Tip of the day - Avoid all-or-nothing thinking. If you aim to exercise for 25 minutes but find you only have 10 minutes, don't feel that because you don't have time for your entire walk or workout you should do nothing. If all you have is 10 minutes, then exercise for 10 minutes. Same with food—don't feel that if you eat one potato chip you have to eat the whole bag. Eat three chips and put the bag away.

taking charge of my health!

eat
- ☐ ate a healthy breakfast
- ☐ had protein at every meal
- ☐ had 1-2 healthy snacks
- ☐ ate dinner by 7:00 p.m.
- ☐ avoided "white" foods
- ☐ drank water or tea instead of sugary drinks

move
- ☐ walked _____ steps/minutes
- ☐ made active choices
- ☐ got other exercise
  _____

choose
- ☐ took my vitamins
- ☐ got enough sleep _____ hrs
- ☐ kept TV time under 2 hours

successes & confessions

rate your attitude today
3 excellent
2 good
1 so-so
0 disaster! plan to do better tomorrow

what I ate today
circle the number of servings

fruit
0 1 2 3 **4**

vegetables
0 1 2 3 4 **5**

whole grains
0 1 2 3 4 5 **6**

calcium-rich foods
0 1 **2 3**

beans
0 1 2

fish
0 1 2

extra lean poultry or meat
0 1 2

glasses of water
0 1 2 3 4 5 6 **7 8** 9 10

times I ate out of boredom, stress, or habit
0 1 2 3 4 5

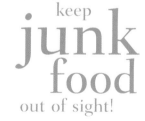

keep
junk
food
out of sight!

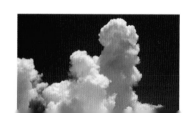

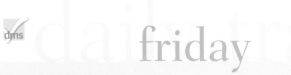

my numbers

weight _____ blood sugar (time/level) _____ / _____ • _____ / _____ • _____ / _____ • _____ / _____

what I ate today

circle the number of servings

fruit

0 1 2 3 **4**

vegetables

0 1 2 3 4 **5**

whole grains

0 1 2 3 4 5 **6**

calcium-rich foods

0 1 **2** **3**

beans

0 1 2

fish

0 1 2

extra lean poultry or meat

0 1 2

glasses of water

0 1 2 3 4 5 6 **7** **8** 9 10

times I ate out of boredom, stress, or habit

0 **1** 2 3 4 5

❋ Tip of the day - Exercise with your spouse. Studies show that couples who start an exercise program together have a higher rate of success than do men or women who exercise without their spouses. If you're single, or if your spouse isn't interested, find an exercise buddy—unhitched exercisers are likely to have similarly high success rates if they team up with a friend.

taking charge of my health!

eat
- ☐ ate a healthy breakfast
- ☐ had protein at every meal
- ☐ had 1-2 healthy snacks
- ☐ ate dinner by 7:00 p.m.
- ☐ avoided "white" foods
- ☐ drank water or tea instead of sugary drinks

move
- ☐ walked _____ steps/minutes
- ☐ made active choices
- ☐ got other exercise

  _____

choose
- ☐ took my vitamins
- ☐ got enough sleep _____ hrs
- ☐ kept TV time under 2 hours

successes & confessions

rate your attitude today

3 excellent
2 good
1 so-so
0 disaster! plan to do better tomorrow

❋ Did you eat a
healthy
breakfast this
morning?

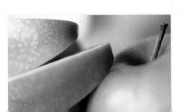

saturday

my numbers

weight _____ blood sugar (time/level) _____ / _____ ⁕ _____ / _____ ⁕ _____ / _____ ⁕ _____ / _____

⁕ Tip of the day - Socialize without food. Who says an outing with friends has to include a trip to the coffee shop, a rich lunch, or a high-calorie dinner? Invite friends on a walk, a hike, a lazy swim in the lake, a visit to a museum, or a game of golf. Activities like these allow you to avoid overeating and burn calories while catching up with friends.

taking charge of my health!

eat
- ☐ ate a healthy breakfast
- ☐ had protein at every meal
- ☐ had 1-2 healthy snacks
- ☐ ate dinner by 7:00 p.m.
- ☐ avoided "white" foods
- ☐ drank water or tea instead of sugary drinks

move
- ☐ walked _____ steps/minutes
- ☐ made active choices
- ☐ got other exercise

_____

choose
- ☐ took my vitamins
- ☐ got enough sleep _____ hrs
- ☐ kept TV time under 2 hours

successes & confessions

rate your attitude today
3 excellent
2 good
1 so-so
0 disaster! plan to do better tomorrow

Did you **stretch** your body today?

what I ate today

circle the number of servings

fruit

0 1 2 3 **4**

vegetables

0 1 2 3 4 **5**

whole grains

0 1 2 3 4 5 **6**

calcium-rich foods

0 1 **2** 3

beans

0 1 2

fish

0 1 2

extra lean poultry or meat

0 1 2

glasses of water

0 1 2 3 4 5 6 **7** **8** 9 10

times I ate out of boredom, stress, or habit

0 **1** 2 3 4 5

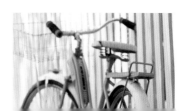

sunday

my numbers

weight _____   blood sugar (time/level) _____ / _____ ⊛ _____ / _____ ⊛ _____ / _____ ⊛ _____ / _____

what I ate today

circle the number of servings

fruit

0 1 2 3 **4**

vegetables

0 1 2 3 4 **5**

whole grains

0 1 2 3 4 5 **6**

calcium-rich foods

0 1 **2** **3**

beans

0 1 2

fish

0 1 2

extra lean poultry or meat

0 1 2

glasses of water

0 1 2 3 4 5 6 **7** **8** 9 10

times I ate out of boredom, stress, or habit

0 **1** 2 3 4 5

✳ **Tip of the day** - Use roasted garlic as a spread for bread in place of butter—you'll add flavor and significantly reduce calories. Cut the tops off two heads of garlic, drizzle with olive oil, wrap in aluminum foil, and roast at 350°F until soft, about an hour. Cool. Squeeze out the garlic, mash, and use on bread or in mashed potatoes.

taking charge of my health!

eat

☐ ate a healthy breakfast
☐ had protein at every meal
☐ had 1-2 healthy snacks
☐ ate dinner by 7:00 p.m.
☐ avoided "white" foods
☐ drank water or tea instead of sugary drinks

move

☐ walked _____ steps/minutes
☐ made active choices
☐ got other exercise

_____

choose

☐ took my vitamins
☐ got enough sleep _____ hrs
☐ kept TV time under 2 hours

successes & confessions

rate your attitude today

3   excellent
2   good
1   so-so
0   disaster! plan to do better tomorrow

Skip the TV tonight and get **active!**

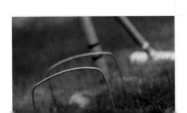

week in review & ahead >

how well I did

eat

Improved my eating
from previous week   *[Yes] [No]*

Made healthy
restaurant choices   *[Yes] [No]*

Tried a new fruit,
vegetable, or grain   *[Yes] [No]*

move

Total walking time _____

Total steps _____
(if using a pedometer)

Walked more than
I did previous week   *[Yes] [No]*

Moved more than
I did previous week   *[Yes] [No]*

Felt more energized
than previous week   *[Yes] [No]*

choose

My attitude this week was:

☐ Positive—I can do this!

☐ Committed—I will follow
   through even if I falter here
   and there

☐ Defeated—need to
   remind myself that every
   little bit counts

Took time for myself   *[Yes] [No]*

Relaxed   *[Yes] [No]*

accomplishments!

_____
_____
_____
_____
_____
_____
_____
_____
_____
_____

☐ Weight loss? _____
☐ Waist measurement: _____
☐ Blood sugar improvement?

_____
_____

"The first wealth
is health."

—Ralph Waldo Emerson

next week's goals

eat It's time to start switching
to whole grains. Buy bread with
the word *whole* in the first
ingredient. Also buy a bag of
brown rice, a bag of barley, and a
box of whole wheat pasta to try.

move Outside of your walks,
look for other opportunities to
move, whether it's taking the
stairs or working on the lawn.
Unless you're sick, don't let
yourself go a day without some
physical activity.

choose As you enter Week
5 of the DMS, keep a can-do attitude. Think of all the ways in
which your health is improving,
and congratulate yourself for all
the progress you've made.

15 ways to say "I love you" without food

For many of us, food means love. We cook up a fattening feast or bake up a person's favorite cookies to demonstrate our appreciation or affection. Or we pick out a beautiful box of chocolates to say "I thought of you." But calorie bombs like these aren't the only way to nurture a relationship. In fact, there are countless ways to express your feelings—and make someone's day.

1 Buy flowers. Just because it's a cliché doesn't mean it won't bring a huge smile to someone's face. You don't have to buy a big bouquet; a single rose or a handful of wildflowers you picked on your way home will absolutely do the trick.

2 Leave a love note. Little notes left in a brown bag lunch or a briefcase mean more than a bag of chips or a brownie. A shirt or jacket pocket is another good place for a thoughtful or romantic message. Or stick a Post-it note on the bathroom or bedroom mirror.

3 Wash the dishes. Or make the bed, clean the car, or vacuum the house. Small acts like these go a long, long way, especially if those aren't usually your chores.

4 Give a massage. Rub your partner's feet or shoulders for five minutes. The happy after-effects will last for hours.

5 Burn a CD or make a tape. Include his favorite songs, or songs with a common theme, such as love, friendship, or happiness.

6 Rent the movie they want to watch. If your husband likes action films, surprise him with one from the video store. If your wife has been wanting to see a recent tearjerker, bring it home unbidden—and watch it with her without complaint.

7 Leave a phone message. Especially if you know someone's having a tough time, leave her a voice message saying "Thinking of you" or "I'm here for you."

8 Write a poem. Just a few lines of verse, rhyming or not, will be a delightful surprise. And penning poetry is a fun challenge.

9 Spend some time. Share a hobby with the grandchildren, invite your kid to play a round of golf, read a book to an elderly parent—it's taking the time and interest that counts.

10 Do what they love to do. If your wife is a gardener, spend the afternoon helping in the garden. If your husband loves to golf, ask him for a golfing lesson. If your parents love art, take them to a crafts show. If your kids love thrills, take them to the amusement park. Nothing shows love better than sharing in a person's pleasures.

11 Fill up your kid's car with gas. It's the unexpected gestures that touch the heart. And if your kid is strapped for cash, this particular gesture will be appreciated doubly.

12 Frame a photo. If you've taken a recent photo of him, her, or the two of you, buy the perfect frame and wrap it up. Most times, the pictures we like sit in piles or boxes. A nice frame makes all the difference.

13 Give a gift certificate for a new pair of sneakers. You'll show you care about his health and want to keep him around as long as possible.

14 Do something thoughtful. Throw a bath towel into the dryer so it's warm when your loved one comes out of the shower, or meet her at the car door with an umbrella when it's raining.

15 Say "I love you." It's the obvious answer, but most of us simply don't say it enough.

weekly meal planner

	Monday	Tuesday	Wednesday
breakfast			
lunch			
dinner			

Higher in protein and lower in saturated fat than either beef or pork, chicken breast is one of the best foods to use as the center of your meal. Plan at least one chicken-breast meal this week. Cook extra chicken and use it the next day to top a salad or include in a sandwich.

When cooking chicken, make sure to remove the skin, where most of the fat is. If you're roasting a chicken, either cook the vegetables separately so they don't soak up all the fat from the chicken, or wait until you've skimmed the fat from the meat juices before adding the vegetables.

For sandwiches, choose roasted turkey, which is even lower in calories than chicken.

Thursday	Friday	Saturday	Sunday

Food Fact One cup of baby carrots has just 35 calories compared with 165 calories for a single ounce of peanuts.

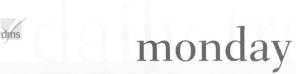

monday

my numbers

weight _____   blood sugar (time/level) _____ / _____ • _____ / _____ • _____ / _____ • _____ / _____

what I ate today

circle the number of servings

fruit

0 1 2 3 **4**

vegetables

0 1 2 3 4 **5**

whole grains

0 1 2 3 4 5 **6**

calcium-rich foods

0 1 **2** **3**

beans

0 1 2

fish

0 1 2

extra lean poultry or meat

0 1 2

glasses of water

0 1 2 3 4 5 6 **7** **8** 9 10

times I ate out of boredom, stress, or habit

0 **1** 2 3 4 5

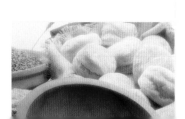

✳ **Tip of the day** - Exercise while you watch TV. Whenever a commercial comes on, get up and walk up and down the stairs, do jumping jacks, or march in place until the program comes back on. Remember: Even small bursts of physical activity add up to weight loss and increased insulin sensitivity.

taking charge of my health!

eat

☐ ate a healthy breakfast

☐ had protein at every meal

☐ had 1-2 healthy snacks

☐ ate dinner by 7:00 p.m.

☐ avoided "white" foods

☐ drank water or tea instead of sugary drinks

move

☐ walked _____ steps/minutes

☐ made active choices

☐ got other exercise

_____

choose

☐ took my vitamins

☐ got enough sleep _____ hrs

☐ kept TV time under 2 hours

successes & confessions

rate your attitude today

3 excellent

2 good

1 so-so

0 disaster! plan to do better tomorrow

Did you eat **whole grain** **breads** today?

tuesday

my numbers

weight _____   blood sugar (time/level) _____ / _____ • _____ / _____ • _____ / _____ • _____ / _____

✳ **Tip of the day** - Move every 30 minutes at work. Set the alarm on your computer or watch to go off every half hour. This is your signal to get up and do a few stretches or take a quick walk. One destination to choose: the water cooler. Water keeps you hydrated, of course, but it can also sometimes stave off a food craving.

taking charge of my health!

eat

☐ ate a healthy breakfast
☐ had protein at every meal
☐ had 1-2 healthy snacks
☐ ate dinner by 7:00 p.m.
☐ avoided "white" foods
☐ drank water or tea instead of sugary drinks

move

☐ walked _____ steps/minutes
☐ made active choices
☐ got other exercise

_____

choose

☐ took my vitamins
☐ got enough sleep _____ hrs
☐ kept TV time under 2 hours

successes & confessions

rate your attitude today

3   excellent
2   good
1   so-so
0   disaster! plan to do better tomorrow

skip the soda
today and
drink
tea or water.

what I ate today

circle the number of servings

fruit

0 1 2 3 **4**

vegetables

0 1 2 3 4 **5**

whole grains

0 1 2 3 4 5 **6**

calcium-rich foods

0 1 **2** **3**

beans

0 1 2

fish

0 1 2

extra lean poultry or meat

0 1 2

glasses of water

0 1 2 3 4 5 6 **7** **8** 9 10

times I ate out of boredom, stress, or habit

0 **1** 2 3 4 5

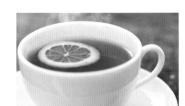

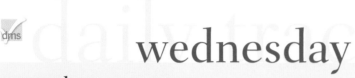

wednesday

my numbers

weight _____ blood sugar (time/level) _____ / _____ • _____ / _____ • _____ / _____ • _____ / _____

what I ate today

circle the number of servings

fruit

0 1 2 3 **4**

vegetables

0 1 2 3 4 **5**

whole grains

0 1 2 3 4 5 **6**

calcium-rich foods

0 1 **2** **3**

beans

0 1 2

fish

0 1 2

extra lean poultry or meat

0 1 2

glasses of water

0 1 2 3 4 5 6 **7** **8** 9 10

times I ate out of boredom, stress, or habit

0 **1** 2 3 4 5

※ **Tip of the day** - When it comes to snacks such as pretzels, peanuts, or popcorn, consider buying individual snack-size packages, even if the big bag is a better value. Studies find that when you buy larger sizes, you eat more. It's just human nature. Limit yourself to one snack-size bag a day.

taking charge of my health!

eat

☐ ate a healthy breakfast

☐ had protein at every meal

☐ had 1-2 healthy snacks

☐ ate dinner by 7:00 p.m.

☐ avoided "white" foods

☐ drank water or tea instead of sugary drinks

move

☐ walked _____ steps/minutes

☐ made active choices

☐ got other exercise

_____

choose

☐ took my vitamins

☐ got enough sleep _____ hrs

☐ kept TV time under 2 hours

successes & confessions

rate your attitude today

3 excellent

2 good

1 so-so

0 disaster! plan to do better tomorrow

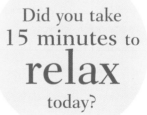

Did you take
15 minutes to
relax
today?

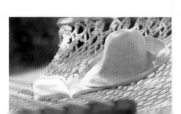

thursday

my numbers

weight _____   blood sugar (time/level) _____ / _____ • _____ / _____ • _____ / _____ • _____ / _____

❋ **Tip of the day** - Do you tend to eat when you're bored? If so, make a list of other things you can in those instances, and post it on your refrigerator. Your list may include calling a friend, taking your dog for a walk, knitting, organizing your photos, or spending time on an old or new hobby.

taking charge of my health!

eat
☐ ate a healthy breakfast
☐ had protein at every meal
☐ had 1-2 healthy snacks
☐ ate dinner by 7:00 p.m.
☐ avoided "white" foods
☐ drank water or tea instead of sugary drinks

move
☐ walked _____ steps/minutes
☐ made active choices
☐ got other exercise
☐ _____

choose
☐ took my vitamins
☐ got enough sleep _____ hrs
☐ kept TV time under 2 hours

successes & confessions

rate your attitude today
3   excellent
2   good
1   so-so
0   disaster! plan to do better tomorrow

what I ate today

circle the number of servings

fruit
0 1 2 3 **4**

vegetables
0 1 2 3 4 **5**

whole grains
0 1 2 3 4 5 **6**

calcium-rich foods
0 1 **2** **3**

beans
0 1 2

fish
0 1 2

extra lean poultry or meat
0 1 2

glasses of water
0 1 2 3 4 5 6 **7** **8** 9 10

times I ate out of boredom, stress, or habit
0 **1** 2 3 4 5

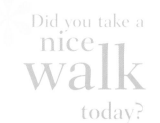

Did you take a
nice
walk
today?

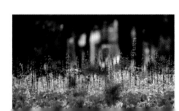

my numbers

weight _____   blood sugar (time/level) _____ / _____ • _____ / _____ • _____ / _____ • _____ / _____

what I ate today

circle the number of servings

fruit

0 1 2 3 **4**

vegetables

0 1 2 3 4 **5**

whole grains

0 1 2 3 4 5 **6**

calcium-rich foods

0 1 **2** **3**

beans

0 1 2

fish

0 1 2

extra lean poultry or meat

0 1 2

glasses of water

0 1 2 3 4 5 6 **7** **8** 9 10

times I ate out of boredom, stress, or habit

0 **1** 2 3 4 5

❊ Tip of the day - Stir-fry your vegetables. It's one of the simplest and healthiest ways to cook. Use a wok if you have one—its small cooking base and wide sides allow you to use less oil (and save on calories) than you would use in a flat-bottomed frying pan. And the fast, high heat used in stir-frying helps preserve food's nutrients, flavor, and crunch.

taking charge of my health!

eat

☐ ate a healthy breakfast
☐ had protein at every meal
☐ had 1-2 healthy snacks
☐ ate dinner by 7:00 p.m.
☐ avoided "white" foods
☐ drank water or tea instead of sugary drinks

move

☐ walked _____ steps/minutes
☐ made active choices
☐ got other exercise

_____

choose

☐ took my vitamins
☐ got enough sleep _____ hrs
☐ kept TV time under 2 hours

successes & confessions

rate your attitude today

3   excellent
2   good
1   so-so
0   disaster! plan to do better tomorrow

Put your fork down between **bites** and eat more slowly.

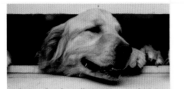

saturday

my numbers

weight _____   blood sugar (time/level) _____ / _____ • _____ / _____ • _____ / _____ • _____ / _____

※ **Tip of the day** - Snack on unsalted peanuts in the shell. The "good" fat in peanuts helps prevent heart disease and keep blood sugar levels steady. Plus, studies show that people who include peanuts in a reduced-calorie diet lose more weight than those who don't. A serving is about 28 peanuts—not much more than a handful. Shelling peanuts while eating them makes a serving last longer.

taking charge of my health!

eat

☐ ate a healthy breakfast
☐ had protein at every meal
☐ had 1-2 healthy snacks
☐ ate dinner by 7:00 p.m.
☐ avoided "white" foods
☐ drank water or tea instead of sugary drinks

move

☐ walked _____ steps/minutes
☐ made active choices
☐ got other exercise

_____

choose

☐ took my vitamins
☐ got enough sleep _____ hrs
☐ kept TV time under 2 hours

successes & confessions

rate your attitude today

3   excellent
2   good
1   so-so
0   disaster! plan to do better
    tomorrow

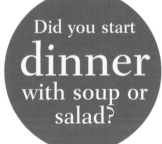

Did you start **dinner** with soup or salad?

what I ate today

circle the number of servings

fruit

0 1 2 3 **4**

vegetables

0 1 2 3 4 **5**

whole grains

0 1 2 3 4 5 **6**

calcium-rich foods

0 1 **2** **3**

beans

0 1 2

fish

0 1 2

extra lean poultry or meat

0 1 2

glasses of water

0 1 2 3 4 5 6 **7** **8** 9 10

times I ate out of boredom, stress, or habit

0 **1** 2 3 4 5

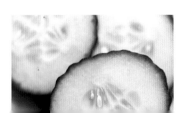

sunday

my numbers

weight _____ blood sugar (time/level) _____ / _____ • _____ / _____ • _____ / _____ • _____ / _____

what I ate today

circle the number of servings

fruit

0 1 2 3 **4**

vegetables

0 1 2 3 4 **5**

whole grains

0 1 2 3 4 5 **6**

calcium-rich foods

0 1 **2** **3**

beans

0 1 2

fish

0 1 2

extra lean poultry or meat

0 1 2

glasses of water

0 1 2 3 4 5 6 **7** **8** 9 10

times I ate out of boredom, stress, or habit

0 **1** 2 3 4 5

※ **Tip of the day** - Exercise after eating. You're less likely to be hit by hypoglycemia if you work out an hour or two after a meal, when your blood sugar will be naturally high and plenty of glucose will be available to fuel your muscles. If this doesn't fit your schedule, plan to work out after a snack.

taking charge of my health!

eat
- ☐ ate a healthy breakfast
- ☐ had protein at every meal
- ☐ had 1-2 healthy snacks
- ☐ ate dinner by 7:00 p.m.
- ☐ avoided "white" foods
- ☐ drank water or tea instead of sugary drinks

rate your attitude today

3   excellent
2   good
1   so-so
0   disaster! plan to do better
    tomorrow

move
- ☐ walked _____ steps/minutes
- ☐ made active choices
- ☐ got other exercise
- _____

choose
- ☐ took my vitamins
- ☐ got enough sleep _____ hrs
- ☐ kept TV time under 2 hours

successes & confessions

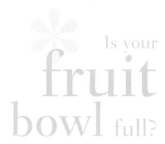

Is your fruit bowl full?

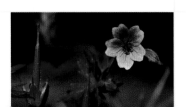

week in review & ahead >

how well I did

eat

Improved my eating
from previous week   *[Yes] [No]*

Made healthy
restaurant choices   *[Yes] [No]*

Tried a new fruit,
vegetable, or grain   *[Yes] [No]*

move

Total walking time _____

Total steps _____
(if using a pedometer)

Walked more than
I did previous week   *[Yes] [No]*

Moved more than
I did previous week   *[Yes] [No]*

Felt more energized
than previous week   *[Yes] [No]*

choose

My attitude this week was:

☐ Positive—I can do this!

☐ Committed—I will follow
     through even if I falter here
     and there

☐ Defeated—need to
     remind myself that every
     little bit counts

Took time for myself   *[Yes] [No]*

Relaxed   *[Yes] [No]*

accomplishments!

_____
_____
_____
_____
_____
_____
_____
_____

☐ Weight loss? _____
☐ Waist measurement: _____
☐ Blood sugar improvement?

_____
_____

“ Happiness is
nothing more than
good health and a
bad memory. ”

—Albert Schweitzer

next week's goals

eat Take aim at fat. The answer
isn't low-fat cookies. It's buying
low-fat or nonfat milk and
yogurt and choosing the leanest
cuts of meat. Find three chicken
breast recipes you like. Avoid
ground beef!

move Crank up your walking
pace a notch. As you speed up,
don't try to lengthen your stride.
Instead, take smaller, more fre-
quent steps. Concentrate on
pumping your arms.

choose Develop a relax-
ation ritual. Sit outside in your
garden for 10 minutes a day. Add
lavender oil to a diffuser and
inhale the scent before you go to
bed. Remember, lowering your
stress hormones can lower your
blood sugar.

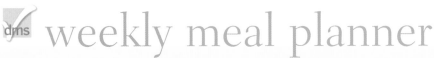

weekly meal planner

date	Monday	Tuesday	Wednesday

When cooking beef, choose round (eye of round, top round, ground round) or loin (tenderloin, sirloin). Flank steak (good for stir-frying) and filet mignon are also lean cuts. When serving beef, make sure to include plenty of vegetables. Sauté beef with peppers and onions, or cook steak pieces in a wok with lots of peppers or broccoli.

If you buy ground beef, don't think that using the fatty kind and pouring off the grease makes it fine. Much of the fat is bound in with the meat. Good quality, 90-percent-or-more ground sirloin is the best choice.

When making beef stew, make it in advance if you can, then chill it and remove the congealed fat before reheating.

breakfast

lunch

dinner

	Thursday	Friday	Saturday	Sunday

Food Fact Dark chocolate contains significantly more antioxidants than milk chocolate—and less fat. Milk chocolate contains milk fat that is highly saturated.

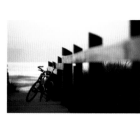

monday

my numbers

weight _____   blood sugar (time/level) _____ / _____ • _____ / _____ • _____ / _____ • _____ / _____

what I ate today

circle the number of servings

fruit

0 1 2 3 **4**

vegetables

0 1 2 3 4 **5**

whole grains

0 1 2 3 4 5 **6**

calcium-rich foods

0 1 **2** **3**

beans

0 1 2

fish

0 1 2

extra lean poultry or meat

0 1 2

glasses of water

0 1 2 3 4 5 6 **7** **8** 9 10

times I ate out of boredom, stress, or habit

0 **1** 2 3 4 5

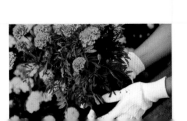

※ Tip of the day - Stay hydrated. Drink a glass of water before and after exercise, and keep a water bottle at hand during your workout to keep yourself from becoming dehydrated. Dehydration can leave you feeling lethargic and too tired to exercise. Don't bother with sugary sports beverages; those are designed for athletes who exercise very vigorously for more than one hour. Most of us don't need the extra calories.

taking charge of my health!

eat

☐ ate a healthy breakfast
☐ had protein at every meal
☐ had 1-2 healthy snacks
☐ ate dinner by 7:00 p.m.
☐ avoided "white" foods
☐ drank water or tea instead of sugary drinks

move

☐ walked _____ steps/minutes
☐ made active choices
☐ got other exercise

_____

choose

☐ took my vitamins
☐ got enough sleep _____ hrs
☐ kept TV time under 2 hours

successes & confessions

rate your attitude today

3 excellent
2 good
1 so-so
0 disaster! plan to do better tomorrow

※ Did you go
somewhere
green
today?

tuesday

my numbers

weight _____ blood sugar (time/level) _____ / _____ • _____ / _____ • _____ / _____ • _____ / _____

✳ **Tip of the day** - Buy plain yogurt and sweeten it yourself. Yogurt is packed with calcium and is an excellent breakfast or snack, but pre-sweetened yogurts are loaded with sugar, which adds calories and raises blood sugar levels. Flavor nonfat, plain yogurt with chopped fresh fruit, a dash of vanilla extract, a sprinkling of nuts or wheat germ, or crushed whole grain cereal.

taking charge of my health!

eat
- ☐ ate a healthy breakfast
- ☐ had protein at every meal
- ☐ had 1-2 healthy snacks
- ☐ ate dinner by 7:00 p.m.
- ☐ avoided "white" foods
- ☐ drank water or tea instead of sugary drinks

move
- ☐ walked _____ steps/minutes
- ☐ made active choices
- ☐ got other exercise

_____

choose
- ☐ took my vitamins
- ☐ got enough sleep _____ hrs
- ☐ kept TV time under 2 hours

successes & confessions

rate your attitude today
3 excellent
2 good
1 so-so
0 disaster! plan to do better tomorrow

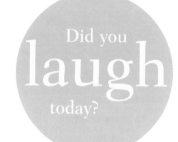
Did you **laugh** today?

what I ate today

circle the number of servings

fruit
0 1 2 3 **4**

vegetables
0 1 2 3 4 **5**

whole grains
0 1 2 3 4 5 **6**

calcium-rich foods
0 1 **2** **3**

beans
0 1 2

fish
0 1 2

extra lean poultry or meat
0 1 2

glasses of water
0 1 2 3 4 5 6 **7** **8** 9 10

times I ate out of boredom, stress, or habit
0 **1** 2 3 4 5

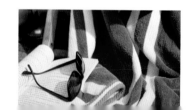

wednesday

my numbers

weight _____   blood sugar (time/level) _____ / _____ ● _____ / _____ ● _____ / _____ ● _____ / _____

what I ate today

circle the number of servings

fruit

0 1 2 3 **4**

vegetables

0 1 2 3 4 **5**

whole grains

0 1 2 3 4 5 **6**

calcium-rich foods

0 1 **2** **3**

beans

0 1 2

fish

0 1 2

extra lean poultry or meat

0 1 2

glasses of water

0 1 2 3 4 5 6 **7** **8** 9 10

times I ate out of boredom, stress, or habit

0 **1** 2 3 4 5

✳ **Tip of the day** - Write down every morsel of food you eat for one week, along with where you ate and what you were doing and feeling at the time. This will help you find patterns that reveal whether, when, and why you overeat—for example, you may notice that you eat too much when you are nervous or overtired.

taking charge of my health!

eat

☐ ate a healthy breakfast

☐ had protein at every meal

☐ had 1-2 healthy snacks

☐ ate dinner by 7:00 p.m.

☐ avoided "white" foods

☐ drank water or tea instead of sugary drinks

move

☐ walked _____ steps/minutes

☐ made active choices

☐ got other exercise

_____

choose

☐ took my vitamins

☐ got enough sleep _____ hrs

☐ kept TV time under 2 hours

rate your attitude today

3 excellent

2 good

1 so-so

0 disaster! plan to do better tomorrow

✳ Keep **junk** food out of sight!

successes & confessions

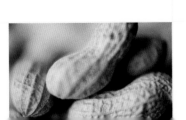

thursday

my numbers

weight _____ blood sugar (time/level) _____ / _____ ∘ _____ / _____ ∘ _____ / _____ ∘ _____ / _____

※ Tip of the day - When adding ground beef to chili, tacos, or meat sauce, buy the leanest grade, brown the meat in a nonstick pan, drain the fat, then rinse the beef with hot water before adding it to your sauce or chili. The water washes away some of the calorie-laden saturated fat that would otherwise go into your recipe.

taking charge of my health!

eat

☐ ate a healthy breakfast
☐ had protein at every meal
☐ had 1-2 healthy snacks
☐ ate dinner by 7:00 p.m.
☐ avoided "white" foods
☐ drank water or tea instead of sugary drinks

move

☐ walked _____ steps/minutes
☐ made active choices
☐ got other exercise
_____

choose

☐ took my vitamins
☐ got enough sleep _____ hrs
☐ kept TV time under 2 hours

successes & confessions

rate your attitude today

3 excellent
2 good
1 so-so
0 disaster! plan to do better tomorrow

Did you find at least **15 minutes** to **relax** today?

what I ate today

circle the number of servings

fruit
0 1 2 3 **4**

vegetables
0 1 2 3 4 **5**

whole grains
0 1 2 3 4 5 **6**

calcium-rich foods
0 1 **2 3**

beans
0 1 2

fish
0 1 2

extra lean poultry or meat
0 1 2

glasses of water
0 1 2 3 4 5 6 **7 8** 9 10

times I ate out of boredom, stress, or habit
0 1 2 3 4 5

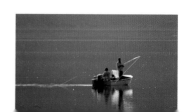

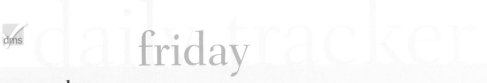

my numbers

weight _____   blood sugar (time/level) _____ / _____ • _____ / _____ • _____ / _____ • _____ / _____

what I ate today

circle the number of servings

fruit

0 1 2 3 **4**

vegetables

0 1 2 3 4 **5**

whole grains

0 1 2 3 4 5 **6**

calcium-rich foods

0 1 **2** **3**

beans

0 1 2

fish

0 1 2

extra lean poultry or meat

0 1 2

glasses of water

0 1 2 3 4 5 6 **7** **8** 9 10

times I ate out of boredom, stress, or habit

0 **1** 2 3 4 5

✻ Tip of the day - Squeeze in exercise throughout the day by taking the stairs instead of the elevator, walking to your neighbor's house to talk instead of phoning, riding your bicycle to do errands instead of driving, and mowing your lawn instead of paying a neighborhood teen to do it. Movement should be an ongoing part of your day.

taking charge of my health!

eat

☐ ate a healthy breakfast
☐ had protein at every meal
☐ had 1-2 healthy snacks
☐ ate dinner by 7:00 p.m.
☐ avoided "white" foods
☐ drank water or tea instead of sugary drinks

move

☐ walked _____ steps/minutes
☐ made active choices
☐ got other exercise

_____

choose

☐ took my vitamins
☐ got enough sleep _____ hrs
☐ kept TV time under 2 hours

successes & confessions

rate your attitude today

3 excellent
2 good
1 so-so
0 disaster! plan to do better tomorrow

Did you **drink enough** **water** today?

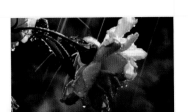

saturday

my numbers

weight _____ blood sugar (time/level) _____ / _____ • _____ / _____ • _____ / _____ • _____ / _____

✳ **Tip of the day** - Discover fresh herbs. Add flavor to vegetables, salads, meat, poultry, and fish with fresh herbs such as basil, rosemary, parsley, oregano, and cilantro. Most grocery stores carry fresh herbs—or grow your own on a sunny windowsill. Be sure to cut herbs with scissors, rather than a knife, to release the most flavor. Store them in the fridge in a glass of water and cover with a plastic bag.

taking charge of my health!

eat
- ☐ ate a healthy breakfast
- ☐ had protein at every meal
- ☐ had 1-2 healthy snacks
- ☐ ate dinner by 7:00 p.m.
- ☐ avoided "white" foods
- ☐ drank water or tea instead of sugary drinks

move
- ☐ walked _____ steps/minutes
- ☐ made active choices
- ☐ got other exercise
  _____

choose
- ☐ took my vitamins
- ☐ got enough sleep _____ hrs
- ☐ kept TV time under 2 hours

successes & confessions

rate your attitude today
3   excellent
2   good
1   so-so
0   disaster! plan to do better tomorrow

Have you checked your **feet** for injuries?

what I ate today
circle the number of servings

fruit
0 1 2 3 **4**

vegetables
0 1 2 3 4 **5**

whole grains
0 1 2 3 4 5 **6**

calcium-rich foods
0 1 **2** 3

beans
0 1 2

fish
0 1 2

extra lean poultry or meat
0 1 2

glasses of water
0 1 2 3 4 5 6 **7 8** 9 10

times I ate out of boredom, stress, or habit
0 1 2 3 4 5

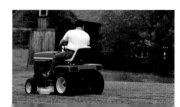

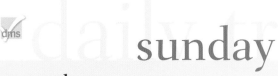
sunday

my numbers

weight _____ blood sugar (time/level) _____ / _____ • _____ / _____ • _____ / _____ • _____ / _____

what I ate today

circle the number of servings

fruit

0 1 2 3 **4**

vegetables

0 1 2 3 4 **5**

whole grains

0 1 2 3 4 5 **6**

calcium-rich foods

0 1 **2** 3

beans

0 1 2

fish

0 1 2

extra lean poultry or meat

0 1 2

glasses of water

0 1 2 3 4 5 6 **7** **8** 9 10

times I ate out of boredom, stress, or habit

0 **1** 2 3 4 5

✳ **Tip of the day** - Follow the 100/100 rule. Eat 100 fewer calories a day (the amount in half a candy bar) and burn 100 more calories a day (by walking 15-20 minutes) and you'll lose almost half a pound a week, or 20 pounds a year. It's not fast, but it's easy and it's definitely significant.

taking charge of my health!

eat

☐ ate a healthy breakfast
☐ had protein at every meal
☐ had 1-2 healthy snacks
☐ ate dinner by 7:00 p.m.
☐ avoided "white" foods
☐ drank water or tea instead of sugary drinks

rate your attitude today

3 excellent
2 good
1 so-so
0 disaster! plan to do better tomorrow

move

☐ walked _____ steps/minutes
☐ made active choices
☐ got other exercise

_____

choose

☐ took my vitamins
☐ got enough sleep _____ hrs
☐ kept TV time under 2 hours

Try a
new
vegetable
this week.

successes & confessions

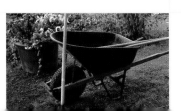

week in review & ahead >

how well I did

eat

Improved my eating
from previous week *[Yes] [No]*

Made healthy
restaurant choices *[Yes] [No]*

Tried a new fruit,
vegetable, or grain *[Yes] [No]*

move

Total walking time _____

Total steps _____
(if using a pedometer)

Walked more than
I did previous week *[Yes] [No]*

Moved more than
I did previous week *[Yes] [No]*

Felt more energized
than previous week *[Yes] [No]*

choose

My attitude this week was:

☐ Positive—I can do this!

☐ Committed—I will follow
through even if I falter here
and there

☐ Defeated—need to
remind myself that every
little bit counts

Took time for myself *[Yes] [No]*

Relaxed *[Yes] [No]*

accomplishments!

_____
_____
_____
_____
_____
_____
_____
_____
_____
_____

☐ Weight loss? _____
☐ Waist measurement: _____
☐ Blood sugar improvement?

_____
_____

" Health is the thing
that makes you feel
that now is the best
time of the year. "

—Franklin P. Adams

next week's goals

eat Zero in on portion sizes,
especially when you're eating
meat. Remember, a dinner serving of meat is just the size of a
deck of cards. Fill the rest of your
plate with veggies and a starch or
a serving of whole grains.

move Plan one activity that
involves being active. Sign up for
a tennis lesson, schedule a short
hike with the family, or test out
the pool at the local YMCA. If
you find a type of exercise you
enjoy, you'll do it more often.

choose Ask your doctor
about supplements such as the
ones in the DMS Supplement
Guide. If nothing else, be sure to
take your multivitamin every day.

13 ways to instantly *improve your* attitude

With the Diabetes Management System, keeping a positive attitude is critical. The right outlook will help you eat better, stick to your walking goals, sleep more soundly, and be more energetic. But everyone feels down or defeated at times. When that happens, turn your attitude around with these simple strategies.

1 Force a smile.
Studies show that the physical act of smiling—even if you don't really mean it—causes chemical changes in your body associated with happiness.

2 Go for a walk.
Exercise triggers the release of feel-good hormones called endorphins. And a dose of fresh air and sunshine never hurt anyone's attitude.

3 Count your blessings.
Write down 5 or 10 things that make you happy or thankful—friends, a beloved pet, a roof over your head, a sunny day— and reflect on each of them for a minute.

4 Picture a soothing scene.
Close your eyes and imagine a scene that's deeply pleasing to you. Perhaps it's a beautiful beach at sunset. Give your full attention to the softness of the sand, the crashing of the waves, the twinkle of the water, and the smell of the salt air.

dms

5 Sniff a scent.
Scents have an amazing impact on your mood. Sprinkle a few drops of an essential oil such as lavender, ylang-ylang, eucalyptus, sandalwood, or rose on a tissue or handkerchief and inhale the scent. If you don't have any essential oil, sniff a flower, light a scented candle, or brew a cup of peppermint tea and breathe in the steam.

6 Put on a great song.
Whether it's soothing classical music, soulful blues, razzy jazz, or rousing rock and roll, music can change your mood faster than you can say "feeling groovy" or "here comes the sun."

7 Get a massage.
Massages not only relieve muscle tension, they trigger the release of serotonin, a brain chemical associated with a feeling of well-being, and reduce levels of the stress hormone cortisol. Bonus: Lowering your stress hormones may even lower your blood sugar. If you can't get a massage from a professional, ask your partner to rub your shoulders for a few minutes, or rub your own feet.

8 See molehills, not mountains. When something goes wrong, ask yourself whether it's really a big deal. Will you remember it years from now? What's the worst thing that can happen as a result? Is it likely to happen?

9 Think of your children or your pet.
Sometimes diverting your thoughts momentarily to those who love you, who matter more, who bring you pleasure, helps you instantly put things in perspective during very stressful moments.

10 Play with a dog.
Playing with a dog for just a few minutes raises levels of the brain chemicals serotonin and oxytocin—both mood elevators. You don't need to own a dog to experience these feel-good effects. Your neighbor's dog would probably love the attention. Or stop by your local pet store. Who knows—you may even end up taking a pooch or kitty home.

11 Find the humor.
When something frustrating happens, think about it as if it happened to someone else—someone you like, or maybe someone you don't. In fact, keep running through the Rolodex in your head until you find the best person you can think of to put in your current predicament. Laugh at him, then laugh at yourself!

12 Put a stop sign in your brain.
When you catch yourself in the midst of negative thinking, shout, "Stop!" to yourself and picture a stop sign. Replace the distressing thought with another thought that's more positive and rational. For example, if the stressful thought is, "I can't do this; I'm worthless," instead say to yourself, "There are many valuable things I can do."

13 Buy yourself flowers.
If you'd buy them for someone else, why not for yourself? You're worth it! Display them on your desk or table to put a little joy in your heart.

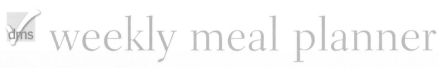

weekly meal planner

date	Monday	Tuesday	Wednesday

Use prepared or packaged foods to give yourself a head start on dinner. Buy marinated chicken breasts. Top frozen pizza crust with plenty of vegetables and low-fat cheese for a fast meal.

Open a bag of frozen vegetables and stir-fry with some quick-peel shrimp for a low-cal dinner, or sauté in a little olive oil and add to pasta along with a little bit of Parmesan cheese for an easy pasta pri-mavera. (Add leftover sliced chicken breast for a heartier meal.)

Cook frozen veggie burgers and top with sliced tomato, onion, mustard, lettuce, salsa, or low-fat feta cheese.

breakfast

lunch

dinner

Thursday	Friday	Saturday	Sunday

Food Fact One slice of American cheese contains 79 calories. Leave the cheese off your sandwich every day for a year and you'll lose 8 pounds.

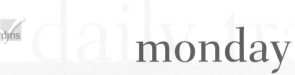
monday

my numbers

weight _____   blood sugar (time/level) _____ / _____ • _____ / _____ • _____ / _____ • _____ / _____

what I ate today

circle the number of servings

fruit

0 1 2 3 **4**

vegetables

0 1 2 3 4 **5**

whole grains

0 1 2 3 4 5 **6**

calcium-rich foods

0 1 **2** **3**

beans

0 1 2

fish

0 1 2

extra lean poultry or meat

0 1 2

glasses of water

0 1 2 3 4 5 6 **7** **8** 9 10

times I ate out of boredom, stress, or habit

0 **1** 2 3 4 5

✳ **Tip of the day** - Forgive yourself. If you make a mistake—you gobble up a huge serving of cherry pie, for example, or you skip your daily walk and go out for ice cream instead—forgive yourself, try to learn from your mistake, and move on. Berating yourself won't help, but resolving to do better next time will.

taking charge of my health!

eat

☐ ate a healthy breakfast

☐ had protein at every meal

☐ had 1-2 healthy snacks

☐ ate dinner by 7:00 p.m.

☐ avoided "white" foods

☐ drank water or tea instead of sugary drinks

move

☐ walked _____ steps/minutes

☐ made active choices

☐ got other exercise

_____

choose

☐ took my vitamins

☐ got enough sleep _____ hrs

☐ kept TV time under 2 hours

rate your attitude today

3   excellent

2   good

1   so-so

0   disaster! plan to do better tomorrow

Is your fridge **stocked with** **healthy** snacks?

successes & confessions

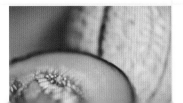

tuesday

my numbers

weight _____ blood sugar (time/level) _____ / _____ • _____ / _____ • _____ / _____ • _____ / _____

☀ **Tip of the day** - Burn calories while you chat. If you spend a lot of time on the phone, invest in a cordless telephone and a headset. Hook the phone onto your back pocket, put on the headset, and get moving. As you catch up with friends or family, you can water houseplants, straighten up the living room, wash windows, or walk on your treadmill if you have one.

taking charge of my health!

eat
☐ ate a healthy breakfast
☐ had protein at every meal
☐ had 1-2 healthy snacks
☐ ate dinner by 7:00 p.m.
☐ avoided "white" foods
☐ drank water or tea instead of sugary drinks

move
☐ walked _____ steps/minutes
☐ made active choices
☐ got other exercise
_____

choose
☐ took my vitamins
☐ got enough sleep _____ hrs
☐ kept TV time under 2 hours

successes & confessions

rate your attitude today
3 excellent
2 good
1 so-so
0 disaster! plan to do better tomorrow

what I ate today
circle the number of servings

fruit
0 1 2 3 **4**

vegetables
0 1 2 3 4 **5**

whole grains
0 1 2 3 4 5 **6**

calcium-rich foods
0 1 **2** **3**

beans
0 1 2

fish
0 1 2

extra lean poultry or meat
0 1 2

glasses of water
0 1 2 3 4 5 6 **7** **8** 9 10

times I ate out of boredom, stress, or habit
0 **1** 2 3 4 5

Keep portion **sizes** in check!

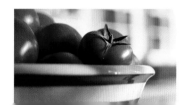

wednesday

my numbers

weight _____ blood sugar (time/level) _____ / _____ • _____ / _____ • _____ / _____ • _____ / _____

what I ate today

circle the number of servings

fruit
0 1 2 3 **4**

vegetables
0 1 2 3 4 **5**

whole grains
0 1 2 3 4 5 **6**

calcium-rich foods
0 1 **2** **3**

beans
0 1 2

fish
0 1 2

extra lean poultry or meat
0 1 2

glasses of water
0 1 2 3 4 5 6 **7 8** 9 10

times I ate out of boredom, stress, or habit
0 1 2 3 4 5

※ Tip of the day - Exercise with a friend. Your walk, jog, or swim will be much more enjoyable—and probably longer—if you go with a companion. Also, a friend can be a great motivator: You're much less likely to skip a workout if you know your buddy is waiting for you.

taking charge of my health!

eat
☐ ate a healthy breakfast
☐ had protein at every meal
☐ had 1-2 healthy snacks
☐ ate dinner by 7:00 p.m.
☐ avoided "white" foods
☐ drank water or tea instead of sugary drinks

move
☐ walked _____ steps/minutes
☐ made active choices
☐ got other exercise
_____

choose
☐ took my vitamins
☐ got enough sleep _____ hrs
☐ kept TV time under 2 hours

successes & confessions

rate your attitude today
3 excellent
2 good
1 so-so
0 disaster! plan to do better tomorrow

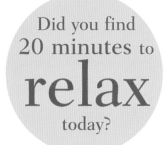
Did you find 20 minutes to relax today?

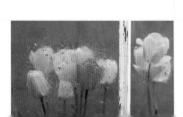

thursday

my numbers

weight _____ blood sugar (time/level) _____ / _____ ● _____ / _____ ● _____ / _____ ● _____ / _____

✳ **Tip of the day** - Leave peels on. Unpeeled fruits and vegetables contain more filling fiber than those with their skin and membranes removed. Wash or scrub unpeeled produce carefully with warm water before eating to remove dirt and bacteria. If you're concerned about pesticide residue, buy organic produce when you can afford it.

taking charge of my health!

eat

☐ ate a healthy breakfast
☐ had protein at every meal
☐ had 1-2 healthy snacks
☐ ate dinner by 7:00 p.m.
☐ avoided "white" foods
☐ drank water or tea instead of sugary drinks

move

☐ walked _____ steps/minutes
☐ made active choices
☐ got other exercise
_____

choose

☐ took my vitamins
☐ got enough sleep _____ hrs
☐ kept TV time under 2 hours

successes & confessions

rate your attitude today

3 excellent
2 good
1 so-so
0 disaster! plan to do better tomorrow

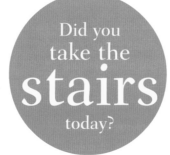

Did you take the **stairs** today?

what I ate today

circle the number of servings

fruit

0 1 2 3 **4**

vegetables

0 1 2 3 4 **5**

whole grains

0 1 2 3 4 5 **6**

calcium-rich foods

0 1 **2 3**

beans

0 1 2

fish

0 1 2

extra lean poultry or meat

0 1 2

glasses of water

0 1 2 3 4 5 6 **7 8** 9 10

times I ate out of boredom, stress, or habit

0 1 2 3 4 5

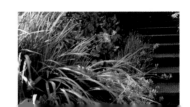

my numbers

weight _____   blood sugar (time/level) _____ / _____ • _____ / _____ • _____ / _____ • _____ / _____

what I ate today

circle the number of servings

fruit
0 1 2 3 **4**

vegetables
0 1 2 3 4 **5**

whole grains
0 1 2 3 4 5 **6**

calcium-rich foods
0 1 **2** 3

beans
0 1 2

fish
0 1 2

extra lean poultry or meat
0 1 2

glasses of water
0 1 2 3 4 5 6 **7 8** 9 10

times I ate out of boredom, stress, or habit
0 1 2 3 4 5

✳ **Tip of the day** - Aim to fill your plate with produce of two or three colors at each meal. Different-colored produce provides different nutrients. For example, dark-green spinach is rich in iron, bright-yellow peppers are full of vitamin C, and rich-red tomatoes contain lycopene, a potent antioxidant.

taking charge of my health!

eat
☐ ate a healthy breakfast
☐ had protein at every meal
☐ had 1-2 healthy snacks
☐ ate dinner by 7:00 p.m.
☐ avoided "white" foods
☐ drank water or tea instead of sugary drinks

move
☐ walked _____ steps/minutes
☐ made active choices
☐ got other exercise
_____

choose
☐ took my vitamins
☐ got enough sleep _____ hrs
☐ kept TV time under 2 hours

successes & confessions

rate your attitude today
3 excellent
2 good
1 so-so
0 disaster! plan to do better tomorrow

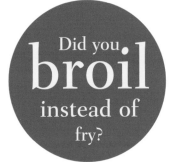

Did you broil instead of fry?

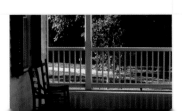

saturday

my numbers

weight _____ blood sugar (time/level) _____ / _____ • _____ / _____ • _____ / _____ • _____ / _____

✳ **Tip of the day** - When recipes call for ground beef, cut the amount in half and bulk up the meat by substituting shredded vegetables, such as onions, carrots, and green peppers, or lower-fat ground turkey or chicken. When buying ground turkey or chicken, choose ground breast, which has fewer calories and less fat than ground poultry that contains a mix of dark and light meat.

taking charge of my health!

eat
☐ ate a healthy breakfast
☐ had protein at every meal
☐ had 1-2 healthy snacks
☐ ate dinner by 7:00 p.m.
☐ avoided "white" foods
☐ drank water or tea instead of sugary drinks

move
☐ walked _____ steps/minutes
☐ made active choices
☐ got other exercise
_____

choose
☐ took my vitamins
☐ got enough sleep _____ hrs
☐ kept TV time under 2 hours

successes & confessions

rate your attitude today
3 excellent
2 good
1 so-so
0 disaster! plan to do better tomorrow

Did you
go somewhere
green
today?

what I ate today
circle the number of servings

fruit
0 1 2 3 **4**

vegetables
0 1 2 3 4 **5**

whole grains
0 1 2 3 4 5 **6**

calcium-rich foods
0 1 **2 3**

beans
0 1 2

fish
0 1 2

extra lean poultry or meat
0 1 2

glasses of water
0 1 2 3 4 5 6 **7 8** 9 10

times I ate out of boredom, stress, or habit
0 1 2 3 4 5

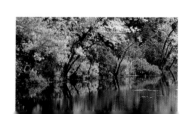

sunday

my numbers

weight _____   blood sugar (time/level) _____ / _____ • _____ / _____ • _____ / _____ • _____ / _____

what I ate today

circle the number of servings

fruit

0 1 2 3 **4**

vegetables

0 1 2 3 4 **5**

whole grains

0 1 2 3 4 5 **6**

calcium-rich foods

0 1 **2** **3**

beans

0 1 2

fish

0 1 2

extra lean poultry or meat

0 1 2

glasses of water

0 1 2 3 4 5 6 **7** **8** 9 10

times I ate out of boredom, stress, or habit

0 **1** 2 3 4 5

※ Tip of the day - Commit to getting plenty of sleep. Studies show that people are more likely to exercise and stick to their eating plan when they are well rested. Aim for seven to eight hours a night, or more if that's what you need to feel fully refreshed. If you need more sleep, move up your bedtime rather than sleeping later in the morning.

taking charge of my health!

eat

☐ ate a healthy breakfast
☐ had protein at every meal
☐ had 1-2 healthy snacks
☐ ate dinner by 7:00 p.m.
☐ avoided "white" foods
☐ drank water or tea instead of sugary drinks

move

☐ walked _____ steps/minutes
☐ made active choices
☐ got other exercise

_____

choose

☐ took my vitamins
☐ got enough sleep _____ hrs
☐ kept TV time under 2 hours

successes & confessions

rate your attitude today

3 excellent
2 good
1 so-so
0 disaster! plan to do better tomorrow

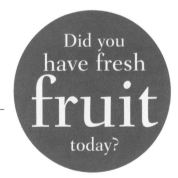
Did you have fresh fruit today?

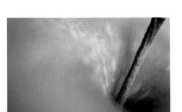

week in review & ahead >

how well I did

eat

Improved my eating
from previous week   [Yes] [No]

Made healthy
restaurant choices   [Yes] [No]

Tried a new fruit,
vegetable, or grain   [Yes] [No]

move

Total walking time _____

Total steps _____
(if using a pedometer)

Walked more than
I did previous week   [Yes] [No]

Moved more than
I did previous week   [Yes] [No]

Felt more energized
than previous week   [Yes] [No]

choose

My attitude this week was:

☐ Positive—I can do this!

☐ Committed—I will follow
   through even if I falter here
   and there

☐ Defeated—need to
   remind myself that every
   little bit counts

Took time for myself   [Yes] [No]

Relaxed   [Yes] [No]

accomplishments!

_____
_____
_____
_____
_____
_____
_____
_____
_____
_____

☐ Weight loss? _____
☐ Waist measurement: _____
☐ Blood sugar improvement?

_____
_____

“He who has health,
has hope. And he
who has hope,
has everything.”

—Arabian Proverb

next week's goals

eat Switch to olive oil and
canola oil, which contain "good"
fats that can help stabilize blood
sugar levels. Use them in place of
butter. Choose extra virgin olive
oil for best taste.

move Starting next week,
your walks should be 30 minutes long. If you're getting
bored with walking, find a new
park to walk through, or explore
a new neighborhood (preferably
a hilly one!).

choose Taking good care of
yourself means taking time for
yourself. Plan to spend at least
three hours next week doing
something you enjoy.

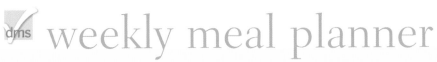

weekly meal planner

date   **Monday**   **Tuesday**   **Wednesday**

breakfast

lunch

dinner

How to get more vegetables into your meals? There are countless ways. First, get in the habit of starting just about every dinner with a green salad.

Sneak chopped vegetables into other foods. Add chopped or pureed carrots to meat loaf. Put chopped or pureed spinach in lasagna or pasta sauce. Add finely chopped mushrooms to beef up burgers.

You can also use vegetables in sauces. Open a jar of herb-seasoned roasted red peppers, puree, and add to tomato sauce or drizzle over fish. Puree butternut or acorn squash with carrots, grated ginger, and a bit of brown sugar for a yummy topping for chicken or turkey.

Thursday	Friday	Saturday	Sunday

Food Fact Some artificial sweeteners break down under high heat, so use brands such as Equal Spoonful or Splenda Granular for baking.

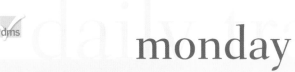

monday

my numbers

weight _____ blood sugar (time/level) _____ / _____ • _____ / _____ • _____ / _____ • _____ / _____

what I ate today

circle the number of servings

fruit

0 1 2 3 **4**

vegetables

0 1 2 3 4 **5**

whole grains

0 1 2 3 4 5 **6**

calcium-rich foods

0 1 **2** **3**

beans

0 1 2

fish

0 1 2

extra lean poultry or meat

0 1 2

glasses of water

0 1 2 3 4 5 6 **7** **8** 9 10

times I ate out of boredom, stress, or habit

0 **1** 2 3 4 5

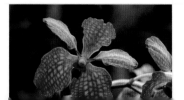

✳ **Tip of the day** - Don't love vegetables? Serve "baby" versions of vegetables such as carrots, spinach and other greens, and brussels sprouts. They tend to have more appealing texture and slightly sweeter flavor. Another tip: Cooking vegetables a little less than usual will change the texture and perhaps even the taste.

taking charge of my health!

eat

☐ ate a healthy breakfast
☐ had protein at every meal
☐ had 1-2 healthy snacks
☐ ate dinner by 7:00 p.m.
☐ avoided "white" foods
☐ drank water or tea instead of sugary drinks

move

☐ walked _____ steps/minutes
☐ made active choices
☐ got other exercise

_____

choose

☐ took my vitamins
☐ got enough sleep _____ hrs
☐ kept TV time under 2 hours

successes & confessions

rate your attitude today

3 excellent
2 good
1 so-so
0 disaster! plan to do better tomorrow

✳ Start your
daywith
a positive
attitude.

tuesday

my numbers

weight _____ blood sugar (time/level) _____ / _____ • _____ / _____ • _____ / _____ • _____ / _____

what I ate today

circle the number of servings

fruit

0 1 2 3 **4**

vegetables

0 1 2 3 4 **5**

whole grains

0 1 2 3 4 5 **6**

calcium-rich foods

0 1 **2 3**

beans

0 1 2

fish

0 1 2

extra lean poultry or meat

0 1 2

glasses of water

0 1 2 3 4 5 6 **7 8** 9 10

times I ate out of boredom, stress, or habit

0 1 2 3 4 5

taking charge of my health!

eat

☐ ate a healthy breakfast
☐ had protein at every meal
☐ had 1-2 healthy snacks
☐ ate dinner by 7:00 p.m.
☐ avoided "white" foods
☐ drank water or tea instead of sugary drinks

move

☐ walked _____ steps/minutes
☐ made active choices
☐ got other exercise
_____

choose

☐ took my vitamins
☐ got enough sleep _____ hrs
☐ kept TV time under 2 hours

rate your attitude today

3 excellent
2 good
1 so-so
0 disaster! plan to do better tomorrow

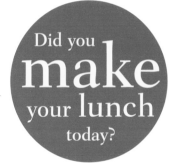

Did you **make** your lunch today?

successes & confessions

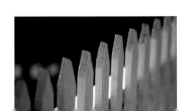

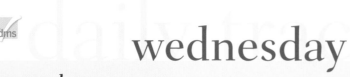

wednesday

my numbers

weight _____ blood sugar (time/level) _____ / _____ • _____ / _____ • _____ / _____ • _____ / _____

what I ate today

circle the number of servings

fruit

0 1 2 3 **4**

vegetables

0 1 2 3 4 **5**

whole grains

0 1 2 3 4 5 **6**

calcium-rich foods

0 1 **2** **3**

beans

0 1 2

fish

0 1 2

extra lean poultry or meat

0 1 2

glasses of water

0 1 2 3 4 5 6 **7** **8** 9 10

times I ate out of boredom, stress, or habit

0 **1** 2 3 4 5

✳ **Tip of the day** - Plan your snacks ahead of time. If you wait until you're starving to select snack foods, you may not choose wisely. After eating your breakfast, decide which healthy snacks you'll eat at mid-morning and mid-afternoon. If you'll be out of the house, pack your snacks and take them with you.

taking charge of my health!

eat

☐ ate a healthy breakfast
☐ had protein at every meal
☐ had 1-2 healthy snacks
☐ ate dinner by 7:00 p.m.
☐ avoided "white" foods
☐ drank water or tea instead of sugary drinks

move

☐ walked _____ steps/minutes
☐ made active choices
☐ got other exercise
_____

choose

☐ took my vitamins
☐ got enough sleep _____ hrs
☐ kept TV time under 2 hours

successes & confessions

rate your attitude today

3 excellent
2 good
1 so-so
0 disaster! plan to do better tomorrow

reward yourself for a recent success.

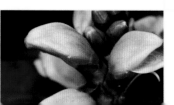

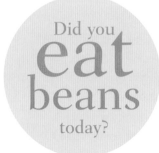

thursday

my numbers

weight _____   blood sugar (time/level) _____ / _____ • _____ / _____ • _____ / _____ • _____ / _____

✳ **Tip of the day** - Once you get in the habit of walking for exercise, you'll want to beef up your walking workouts. One way to do it is by hitting the hills. It burns extra calories but doesn't take any longer than a less intense walk. Find a park or neighborhood street that has ups and downs, and view the inclines as a personal challenge!

taking charge of my health!

eat
☐ ate a healthy breakfast
☐ had protein at every meal
☐ had 1-2 healthy snacks
☐ ate dinner by 7:00 p.m.
☐ avoided "white" foods
☐ drank water or tea instead of sugary drinks

move
☐ walked _____ steps/minutes
☐ made active choices
☐ got other exercise
_____

choose
☐ took my vitamins
☐ got enough sleep _____ hrs
☐ kept TV time under 2 hours

successes & confessions

rate your attitude today
3 excellent
2 good
1 so-so
0 disaster! plan to do better tomorrow

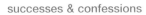

what I ate today
circle the number of servings

fruit
0 1 2 3 **4**

vegetables
0 1 2 3 4 **5**

whole grains
0 1 2 3 4 5 **6**

calcium-rich foods
0 1 **2 3**

beans
0 1 2

fish
0 1 2

extra lean poultry or meat
0 1 2

glasses of water
0 1 2 3 4 5 6 **7 8** 9 10

times I ate out of boredom, stress, or habit
0 1 2 3 4 5

Did you **eat beans** today?

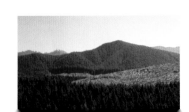

my numbers

weight _____ blood sugar (time/level) _____ / _____ • _____ / _____ • _____ / _____ • _____ / _____

what I ate today

circle the number of servings

fruit

0 1 2 3 **4**

vegetables

0 1 2 3 4 **5**

whole grains

0 1 2 3 4 5 **6**

calcium-rich foods

0 1 **2** **3**

beans

0 1 2

fish

0 1 2

extra lean poultry or meat

0 1 2

glasses of water

0 1 2 3 4 5 6 **7** **8** 9 10

times I ate out of boredom, stress, or habit

0 **1** 2 3 4 5

✳ Tip of the day - Make mealtime relaxing and enjoyable. Serve food on attractive dishes, shut off the television, push aside the newspaper, and let the answering machine pick up your calls. Focus on really tasting your food, rather than rushing through it—people who eat slowly usually eat less than those who speed through their meals.

taking charge of my health!

eat

☐ ate a healthy breakfast

☐ had protein at every meal

☐ had 1-2 healthy snacks

☐ ate dinner by 7:00 p.m.

☐ avoided "white" foods

☐ drank water or tea instead of sugary drinks

move

☐ walked _____ steps/minutes

☐ made active choices

☐ got other exercise

_____

choose

☐ took my vitamins

☐ got enough sleep _____ hrs

☐ kept TV time under 2 hours

successes & confessions

rate your attitude today

3 excellent

2 good

1 so-so

0 disaster! plan to do better tomorrow

*Plan
your meals
for the week.

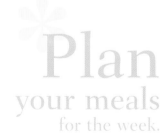

saturday

my numbers

weight _____ blood sugar (time/level) _____ / _____ • _____ / _____ • _____ / _____ • _____ / _____

✳ Tip of the day - Have a goal. Exercise is more fun when you're working toward something specific. Sign up for a charity walk, a 5K run, or a golf tournament. Or keep track of how much time you spend exercising and treat yourself to a massage or a new CD for your portable stereo when you reach, say, 500 minutes of exercise.

taking charge of my health!

eat

☐ ate a healthy breakfast
☐ had protein at every meal
☐ had 1-2 healthy snacks
☐ ate dinner by 7:00 p.m.
☐ avoided "white" foods
☐ drank water or tea instead of sugary drinks

move

☐ walked _____ steps/minutes
☐ made active choices
☐ got other exercise
_____

choose

☐ took my vitamins
☐ got enough sleep _____ hrs
☐ kept TV time under 2 hours

successes & confessions

rate your attitude today

3 excellent
2 good
1 so-so
0 disaster! plan to do better tomorrow

Don't eat **eat** out of **boredom.**

what I ate today

circle the number of servings

fruit
0 1 2 3 **4**

vegetables
0 1 2 3 4 **5**

whole grains
0 1 2 3 4 5 **6**

calcium-rich foods
0 1 **2 3**

beans
0 1 2

fish
0 1 2

extra lean poultry or meat
0 1 2

glasses of water
0 1 2 3 4 5 6 **7 8** 9 10

times I ate out of boredom, stress, or habit
0 1 2 3 4 5

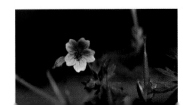

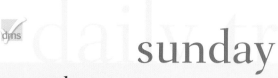

sunday

my numbers

weight _____ blood sugar (time/level) _____ / _____ • _____ / _____ • _____ / _____ • _____ / _____

what I ate today

circle the number of servings

fruit

0 1 2 3 **4**

vegetables

0 1 2 3 4 **5**

whole grains

0 1 2 3 4 5 **6**

calcium-rich foods

0 1 **2** **3**

beans

0 1 2

fish

0 1 2

extra lean poultry or meat

0 1 2

glasses of water

0 1 2 3 4 5 6 **7** **8** 9 10

times I ate out of boredom, stress, or habit

0 **1** 2 3 4 5

※ **Tip of the day** - Drink a tall glass of water with dinner. Between each bite, put down your fork and take a small sip of water—it will make you slow down. Water also helps fill you up and cleanses your palate, allowing you to taste flavors fully.

taking charge of my health!

eat

☐ ate a healthy breakfast

☐ had protein at every meal

☐ had 1-2 healthy snacks

☐ ate dinner by 7:00 p.m.

☐ avoided "white" foods

☐ drank water or tea instead of sugary drinks

move

☐ walked _____ steps/minutes

☐ made active choices

☐ got other exercise

_____

choose

☐ took my vitamins

☐ got enough sleep _____ hrs

☐ kept TV time under 2 hours

rate your attitude today

3 excellent

2 good

1 so-so

0 disaster! plan to do better tomorrow

※ Try a new
grain
this week.

successes & confessions

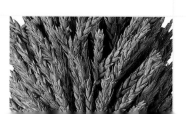

week in review & ahead >

how well I did

eat

Improved my eating
from previous week   *[Yes] [No]*

Made healthy
restaurant choices   *[Yes] [No]*

Tried a new fruit,
vegetable, or grain   *[Yes] [No]*

move

Total walking time _____

Total steps _____
(if using a pedometer)

Walked more than
I did previous week   *[Yes] [No]*

Moved more than
I did previous week   *[Yes] [No]*

Felt more energized
than previous week   *[Yes] [No]*

choose

My attitude this week was:

☐ Positive—I can do this!

☐ Committed—I will follow
   through even if I falter here
   and there

☐ Defeated—need to
   remind myself that every
   little bit counts

Took time for myself   *[Yes] [No]*

Relaxed   *[Yes] [No]*

accomplishments!

_____
_____
_____
_____
_____
_____
_____
_____
_____

☐ Weight loss? _____
☐ Waist measurement: _____
☐ Blood sugar improvement?

_____
_____

" Take care of
your body. It's the only
place you have
to live. "

—Jim Rohn

next week's goals

eat Stock up on smart snacks.
Remember, you should be snacking twice a day—but healthy
snacking requires some prepara-
tion. Have on hand nuts, fresh
fruit, cut-up raw vegetables, and
low-fat yogurt.

move Make use of your time
in front of the TV. Walk on your
treadmill or, if you don't have
one, do arm circles or march in
place during the commercials.

choose Practice waiting
until you're truly hungry to eat.
If there's just one food you want
(especially if it's something sweet
or greasy), it's a craving, not
hunger. Go for a walk instead.

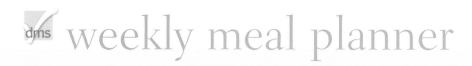

weekly meal planner

date	Monday	Tuesday	Wednesday

Many of us just aren't used to eating fish. But it's fast and easy to cook, in addition to being good for you, so we think you'll get "hooked" once you try it. Aim to eat fish twice a week. Broil it under the broiler, lightly sauté it in a pan, poach it by simmering it in a bit of broth or wine, or steam it. Try Asian Steamed Fish Fillets with Vegetable Sticks (recipe card attached).

Shrimp, which once had a bad reputation, is actually very low in saturated fat and relatively low in calories. So are scallops. Try Sea Scallop and Cherry Tomato Sauté (recipe card attached).

breakfast

lunch

dinner

Thursday   Friday   Saturday   Sunday

Food Fact A food's glycemic load (GL) indicates the impact
it has on blood sugar All-Bran cereal has a GL of just
9 compared with a GL of 21 for cornflakes. A GL of
20 more is considered high.

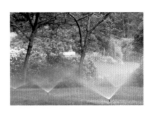

monday

my numbers

weight _____   blood sugar (time/level) _____ / _____ ● _____ / _____ ● _____ / _____ ● _____ / _____

what I ate today

circle the number of servings

fruit
0 1 2 3 **4**

vegetables
0 1 2 3 4 **5**

whole grains
0 1 2 3 4 5 **6**

calcium-rich foods
0 1 **2** 3

beans
0 1 2

fish
0 1 2

extra lean poultry or meat
0 1 2

glasses of water
0 1 2 3 4 5 6 **7 8** 9 10

times I ate out of boredom, stress, or habit
0 1 2 3 4 5

※ **Tip of the day** - Keep sugarless gum everywhere—in your car, purse, briefcase, desk drawer. When you are tempted to eat an unplanned, bad-for-you snack, grab a piece of gum instead. Chewing gum provides a distraction and may buy you time to wait out your junk food craving.

taking charge of my health!

eat
☐ ate a healthy breakfast
☐ had protein at every meal
☐ had 1-2 healthy snacks
☐ ate dinner by 7:00 p.m.
☐ avoided "white" foods
☐ drank water or tea instead of sugary drinks

rate your attitude today
3 excellent
2 good
1 so-so
0 disaster! plan to do better tomorrow

move
☐ walked _____ steps/minutes
☐ made active choices
☐ got other exercise

_____

choose
☐ took my vitamins
☐ got enough sleep _____ hrs
☐ kept TV time under 2 hours

successes & confessions

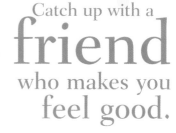

Catch up with a **friend** who makes you feel good.

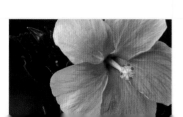

tuesday

my numbers

weight _____   blood sugar (time/level) _____ / _____ • _____ / _____ • _____ / _____ • _____ / _____

✳ **Tip of the day** - Next time you're making meat sauce or chili, substitute soy crumbles for half the beef. Found in the freezer section of natural food or grocery stores, soy crumbles have the texture of meat, and will fool even the meat-lovers in your family, while slashing the amount of saturated fat in your meal.

taking charge of my health!

eat
☐ ate a healthy breakfast
☐ had protein at every meal
☐ had 1-2 healthy snacks
☐ ate dinner by 7:00 p.m.
☐ avoided "white" foods
☐ drank water or tea instead of sugary drinks

move
☐ walked _____ steps/minutes
☐ made active choices
☐ got other exercise
_____

choose
☐ took my vitamins
☐ got enough sleep _____ hrs
☐ kept TV time under 2 hours

successes & confessions

rate your attitude today
3   excellent
2   good
1   so-so
0   disaster! plan to do better tomorrow

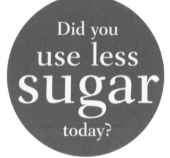
Did you **use less sugar** today?

what I ate today

circle the number of servings

fruit
0 1 2 3 **4**

vegetables
0 1 2 3 4 **5**

whole grains
0 1 2 3 4 5 **6**

calcium-rich foods
0 1 **2 3**

beans
0 1 2

fish
0 1 2

extra lean poultry or meat
0 1 2

glasses of water
0 1 2 3 4 5 6 **7 8** 9 10

times I ate out of boredom, stress, or habit
0 1 2 3 4 5

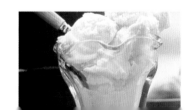

wednesday

my numbers

weight _____   blood sugar (time/level) _____ / _____ • _____ / _____ • _____ / _____ • _____ / _____

what I ate today

circle the number of servings

fruit

0 1 2 3 **4**

vegetables

0 1 2 3 4 **5**

whole grains

0 1 2 3 4 5 **6**

calcium-rich foods

0 1 **2** **3**

beans

0 1 2

fish

0 1 2

extra lean poultry or meat

0 1 2

glasses of water

0 1 2 3 4 5 6 **7** **8** 9 10

times I ate out of boredom, stress, or habit

0 **1** 2 3 4 5

※ **Tip of the day** - Use the talk test. When you exercise, you should push yourself enough that you are breathing faster and your heart is beating harder than usual, but not so hard that you can't catch your breath. If you're too winded to carry on a conversation while exercising, slow down.

taking charge of my health!

eat

☐ ate a healthy breakfast

☐ had protein at every meal

☐ had 1-2 healthy snacks

☐ ate dinner by 7:00 p.m.

☐ avoided "white" foods

☐ drank water or tea instead of sugary drinks

move

☐ walked _____ steps/minutes

☐ made active choices

☐ got other exercise

_____

choose

☐ took my vitamins

☐ got enough sleep _____ hrs

☐ kept TV time under 2 hours

successes & confessions

rate your attitude today

3 excellent

2 good

1 so-so

0 disaster! plan to do better tomorrow

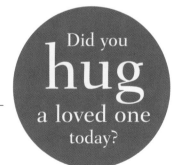
Did you **hug** a loved one today?

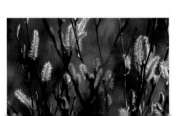

thursday

my numbers

weight _____   blood sugar (time/level) _____ / _____ • _____ / _____ • _____ / _____ • _____ / _____

✳ **Tip of the day** - Drink your milk. Research shows that people whose diets are rich in calcium-containing dairy products such as milk lose more weight and body fat than those whose diets are low in calcium. Just remember to choose nonfat or low-fat dairy products. Taking a calcium supplement is also smart. Buy pills with 600 milligrams of calcium and take one pill twice a day.

taking charge of my health!

eat

☐ ate a healthy breakfast
☐ had protein at every meal
☐ had 1-2 healthy snacks
☐ ate dinner by 7:00 p.m.
☐ avoided "white" foods
☐ drank water or tea instead of sugary drinks

move

☐ walked _____ steps/minutes
☐ made active choices
☐ got other exercise
   _____

choose

☐ took my vitamins
☐ got enough sleep _____ hrs
☐ kept TV time under 2 hours

successes & confessions
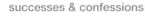

rate your attitude today

3   excellent
2   good
1   so-so
0   disaster! plan to do better tomorrow

what I ate today

circle the number of servings

fruit

0 1 2 3 **4**

vegetables

0 1 2 3 4 **5**

whole grains

0 1 2 3 4 5 **6**

calcium-rich foods

0 1 **2** 3

beans

0 1 2

fish

0 1 2

extra lean poultry or meat

0 1 2

glasses of water

0 1 2 3 4 5 6 **7** **8** 9 10

times I ate out of boredom, stress, or habit

0 **1** 2 3 4 5

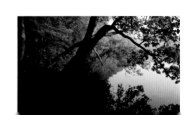

friday

dms daily tracker

my numbers

weight _____ blood sugar (time/level) _____ / _____ • _____ / _____ • _____ / _____ • _____ / _____

what I ate today

circle the number of servings

fruit

0 1 2 3 **4**

vegetables

0 1 2 3 4 **5**

whole grains

0 1 2 3 4 5 **6**

calcium-rich foods

0 1 **2 3**

beans

0 1 2

fish

0 1 2

extra lean poultry or meat

0 1 2

glasses of water

0 1 2 3 4 5 6 **7 8** 9 10

times I ate out of boredom, stress, or habit

0 1 2 3 4 5

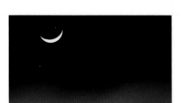

Tip of the day

✳ Tip of the day - When you're eating in a restaurant, look for menu items that include the following healthy-cooking terms: *Baked, braised, blackened, broiled, grilled, poached, roasted, steamed.* Avoid foods that are *fried, breaded, stuffed,* or *crunchy.* And always ask for the sauce or dressing on the side so you can control the amount you eat.

taking charge of my health!

eat

☐ ate a healthy breakfast
☐ had protein at every meal
☐ had 1-2 healthy snacks
☐ ate dinner by 7:00 p.m.
☐ avoided "white" foods
☐ drank water or tea instead of sugary drinks

move

☐ walked _____ steps/minutes
☐ made active choices
☐ got other exercise

_____

choose

☐ took my vitamins
☐ got enough sleep _____ hrs
☐ kept TV time under 2 hours

successes & confessions

rate your attitude today

3 excellent
2 good
1 so-so
0 disaster! plan to do better tomorrow

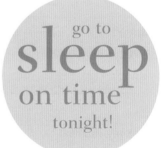

go to **sleep** on time tonight!

saturday

my numbers

weight _____ blood sugar (time/level) _____ / _____ • _____ / _____ • _____ / _____ • _____ / _____

✳ **Tip of the day** - Start dinner with soup or a big salad. Studies show that people who begin a meal with a clear soup (avoid cream-based soups) or green salad consume fewer calories overall at the meal. Soups and salads fill you up without a lot of calories.

taking charge of my health!

eat
- ☐ ate a healthy breakfast
- ☐ had protein at every meal
- ☐ had 1-2 healthy snacks
- ☐ ate dinner by 7:00 p.m.
- ☐ avoided "white" foods
- ☐ drank water or tea instead of sugary drinks

move
- ☐ walked _____ steps/minutes
- ☐ made active choices
- ☐ got other exercise
- _____

choose
- ☐ took my vitamins
- ☐ got enough sleep _____ hrs
- ☐ kept TV time under 2 hours

successes & confessions

rate your attitude today
3 excellent
2 good
1 so-so
0 disaster! plan to do better tomorrow

what I ate today

circle the number of servings

fruit

0 1 2 3 **4**

vegetables

0 1 2 3 4 **5**

whole grains

0 1 2 3 4 5 **6**

calcium-rich foods

0 1 **2** 3

beans

0 1 2

fish

0 1 2

extra lean poultry or meat

0 1 2

glasses of water

0 1 2 3 4 5 6 **7** **8** 9 10

times I ate out of boredom, stress, or habit

0 **1** 2 3 4 5

keep junk food out of sight

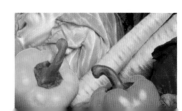

sunday

my numbers

weight _____   blood sugar (time/level) _____ / _____ • _____ / _____ • _____ / _____ • _____ / _____

what I ate today

circle the number of servings

fruit

0 1 2 3 **4**

vegetables

0 1 2 3 4 **5**

whole grains

0 1 2 3 4 5 **6**

calcium-rich foods

0 1 **2** 3

beans

0 1 2

fish

0 1 2

extra lean poultry or meat

0 1 2

glasses of water

0 1 2 3 4 5 6 **7** **8** 9 10

times I ate out of boredom, stress, or habit

0 **1** 2 3 4 5

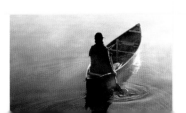

Tip of the day

❋ Tip of the day - Take a chicken breast holiday. It's an excellent weight-loss food, but it can get boring. The next time you pull out that same old chicken breast recipe, replace the chicken with other lean choices: salmon, turkey breast, pork tenderloin, firm tofu, beef tenderloin, or even cashews.

taking charge of my health!

eat

☐ ate a healthy breakfast
☐ had protein at every meal
☐ had 1-2 healthy snacks
☐ ate dinner by 7:00 p.m.
☐ avoided "white" foods
☐ drank water or tea instead of sugary drinks

move

☐ walked _____ steps/minutes
☐ made active choices
☐ got other exercise

_____

choose

☐ took my vitamins
☐ got enough sleep _____ hrs
☐ kept TV time under 2 hours

successes & confessions

rate your attitude today

3 excellent
2 good
1 so-so
0 disaster! plan to do better tomorrow

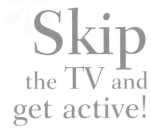

Skip the TV and get active!

week in review & ahead >

how well I did

eat

Improved my eating
from previous week   *[Yes] [No]*

Made healthy
restaurant choices   *[Yes] [No]*

Tried a new fruit,
vegetable, or grain   *[Yes] [No]*

move

Total walking time _____

Total steps _____
(if using a pedometer)

Walked more than
I did previous week   *[Yes] [No]*

Moved more than
I did previous week   *[Yes] [No]*

Felt more energized
than previous week   *[Yes] [No]*

choose

My attitude this week was:

☐ Positive—I can do this!

☐ Committed—I will follow
through even if I falter here
and there

☐ Defeated—need to
remind myself that every
little bit counts

Took time for myself   *[Yes] [No]*

Relaxed   *[Yes] [No]*

accomplishments!

_____
_____
_____
_____
_____
_____
_____
_____
_____

☐ Weight loss? _____
☐ Waist measurement: _____
☐ Blood sugar improvement?

_____
_____

" You can set
yourself up to be sick,
or you can choose to
stay well. "

—Wayne Dyer

next week's goals

eat Eat fish or shellfish twice
next week. Fresh fish is best
eaten the day you buy it, but it
will keep for up to a day or two
if kept very cold.

move Building up your muscles is important for diabetes. To
work your upper body, do wall
push-ups (like regular push-ups
but standing up and pressing
against a wall) every day next
week. Try to add two push-ups
every day.

choose Banish negative
thoughts. When you have a negative thought, write it down,
then write down a more positive
version of the same thought and
choose to believe it.

15 delicious snacks

dms

1. 1 cup sliced, raw vegetables such as carrots or red peppers
40 CALORIES

2. 1 apple
80 CALORIES

3. 1 ounce fat-free string cheese
80 CALORIES

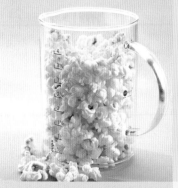

4. 4 cups air-popped popcorn,
100 CALORIES

5. 1 celery stick with 1 tablespoon of peanut butter
85 CALORIES

6. 1 handful pumpkin or sunflower seeds
90 CALORIES

7. 1 cup nonfat yogurt, with 1/2 cup strawberries
150 CALORIES

8. Hard-boiled egg
80 CALORIES

for stable blood sugar

9.
Frozen fruit bar, no sugar added

25 CALORIES

10.
1 Fudgsicle

80 CALORIES

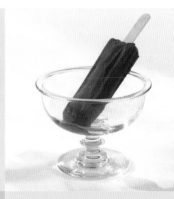

11.
8 ounces tomato juice

40 CALORIES

12.
4 ounces fat-free pudding

100 CALORIES

13.
1/2 cup applesauce

80 CALORIES

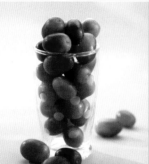

14.
20 red grapes

80 CALORIES

15.
20 Almonds

100 CALORIES

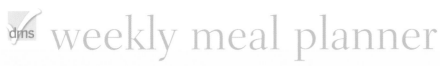

date	Monday	Tuesday	Wednesday

They may not be glamorous, but canned beans are convenient, cheap, and versatile. They are also highly nutritious—and a powerful way to lower your cholesterol. Plan one bean-based dinner this week. Try Chili with White Beans, Tomatoes, and Corn (recipe card attached).

other ways to use beans:

• Spread nonfat refried beans on a whole wheat burrito and sprinkle with chopped chicken and shredded cheese.

• Use a half-cup of black beans and salsa as a filling for your omelet.

• Make a bean salad with canned black beans, fresh or frozen corn kernels, chopped cilantro, chopped onion, and chopped tomato. Drizzle with olive oil and a dash of vinegar, salt, and pepper.

• Stock up on cans of black bean and lentil soup for lunch.

breakfast

lunch

dinner

Thursday	Friday	Saturday	Sunday

Food Fact Studies have shown that coffee can lower blood sugar. It's not the caffeine that does it but other compounds, most likely chlorogenic acids. Decaf is best, since caffeine hampers insulin's effectiveness.

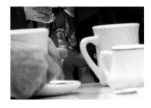

monday

my numbers

weight _____   blood sugar (time/level) _____ / _____ • _____ / _____ • _____ / _____ • _____ / _____

what I ate today

circle the number of servings

fruit

0 1 2 3 **4**

vegetables

0 1 2 3 4 **5**

whole grains

0 1 2 3 4 5 **6**

calcium-rich foods

0 1 **2** **3**

beans

0 1 2

fish

0 1 2

extra lean poultry or meat

0 1 2

glasses of water

0 1 2 3 4 5 6 **7** **8** 9 10

times I ate out of boredom, stress, or habit

0 **1** 2 3 4 5

* Tip of the day - Watch how much juice you drink. Beverages that contain 100% juice contain vitamins—but also plenty of calories. And juice drinks that contain only a little juice are devoid of nutrition. Mix juice with seltzer to stretch it out. And choose fresh fruit over juice whenever you can. It's more filling because it contains fiber, which juice lacks.

taking charge of my health!

eat

☐ ate a healthy breakfast
☐ had protein at every meal
☐ had 1-2 healthy snacks
☐ ate dinner by 7:00 p.m.
☐ avoided "white" foods
☐ drank water or tea instead of sugary drinks

move

☐ walked _____ steps/minutes
☐ made active choices
☐ got other exercise

_____

choose

☐ took my vitamins
☐ got enough sleep _____ hrs
☐ kept TV time under 2 hours

successes & confessions

rate your attitude today

3   excellent
2   good
1   so-so
0   disaster! plan to do better tomorrow

Did you **eat** a healthy breakfast this morning?

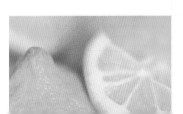

tuesday

my numbers

weight _____ blood sugar (time/level) _____ / _____ • _____ / _____ • _____ / _____ • _____ / _____

✳ **Tip of the day** - Remove temptation when you eat in restaurants by asking the waiter to take away the chips or the bread basket. Chips, bread, and butter add calories and fat. If you're starving when you sit down, ask the waiter to bring you a glass of tomato juice right away.

taking charge of my health!

eat
☐ ate a healthy breakfast
☐ had protein at every meal
☐ had 1-2 healthy snacks
☐ ate dinner by 7:00 p.m.
☐ avoided "white" foods
☐ drank water or tea instead
  of sugary drinks

move
☐ walked _____ steps/minutes
☐ made active choices
☐ got other exercise
  _____

choose
☐ took my vitamins
☐ got enough sleep _____ hrs
☐ kept TV time under 2 hours

successes & confessions

rate your attitude today
3 excellent
2 good
1 so-so
0 disaster! plan to do better
  tomorrow

Did you take at least 15 minutes to **relax** today?

what I ate today

circle the number of servings

fruit
0 1 2 3 **4**

vegetables
0 1 2 3 4 **5**

whole grains
0 1 2 3 4 5 **6**

calcium-rich foods
0 1 **2 3**

beans
0 1 2

fish
0 1 2

extra lean poultry or meat
0 1 2

glasses of water
0 1 2 3 4 5 6 **7 8** 9 10

times I ate out of boredom, stress, or habit
0 1 2 3 4 5

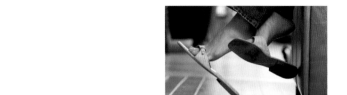

dms

wednesday

my numbers

weight _____ blood sugar (time/level) _____ / _____ • _____ / _____ • _____ / _____ • _____ / _____

what I ate today

circle the number of servings

fruit

0 1 2 3 **4**

vegetables

0 1 2 3 4 **5**

whole grains

0 1 2 3 4 5 **6**

calcium-rich foods

0 1 **2** 3

beans

0 1 2

fish

0 1 2

extra lean poultry or meat

0 1 2

glasses of water

0 1 2 3 4 5 6 **7 8** 9 10

times I ate out of boredom, stress, or habit

0 1 2 3 4 5

✳ **Tip of the day** - Eat less by eating more often. Studies show that having small meals and snacks throughout the day—rather than two or three big meals—helps stabilize blood sugar and lower cholesterol levels. Eating more frequently also keeps your metabolism in high gear. Some researchers estimate that it makes the body burn as much as 10 percent more calories.

taking charge of my health!

eat

☐ ate a healthy breakfast
☐ had protein at every meal
☐ had 1-2 healthy snacks
☐ ate dinner by 7:00 p.m.
☐ avoided "white" foods
☐ drank water or tea instead of sugary drinks

move

☐ walked _____ steps/minutes
☐ made active choices
☐ got other exercise

_____

choose

☐ took my vitamins
☐ got enough sleep _____ hrs
☐ kept TV time under 2 hours

successes & confessions

rate your attitude today

3 excellent
2 good
1 so-so
0 disaster! plan to do better tomorrow

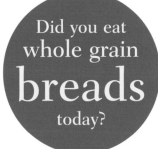
Did you eat **whole grain breads** today?

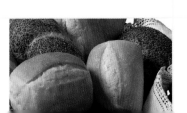

thursday

my numbers

weight _____ blood sugar (time/level) _____ / _____ • _____ / _____ • _____ / _____ • _____ / _____

✳ **Tip of the day** - Set clear, immediate goals that are specific and oriented to what you can actually do, not where you want to end up. For example, it's better to set a goal of "I'll walk five minutes longer next time" than "I want to be able to run five miles by the holidays." Decide that you will eat fruit for dessert twice this week, not that you'll overhaul your entire diet overnight.

taking charge of my health!

eat
☐ ate a healthy breakfast
☐ had protein at every meal
☐ had 1-2 healthy snacks
☐ ate dinner by 7:00 p.m.
☐ avoided "white" foods
☐ drank water or tea instead of sugary drinks

move
☐ walked _____ steps/minutes
☐ made active choices
☐ got other exercise
_____

choose
☐ took my vitamins
☐ got enough sleep _____ hrs
☐ kept TV time under 2 hours

successes & confessions

rate your attitude today
3 excellent
2 good
1 so-so
0 disaster! plan to do better tomorrow

Did you **stretch** your body today?

what I ate today

circle the number of servings

fruit
0 1 2 3 **4**

vegetables
0 1 2 3 4 **5**

whole grains
0 1 2 3 4 5 **6**

calcium-rich foods
0 1 **2 3**

beans
0 1 2

fish
0 1 2

extra lean poultry or meat
0 1 2

glasses of water
0 1 2 3 4 5 6 **7 8** 9 10

times I ate out of boredom, stress, or habit
0 1 2 3 4 5

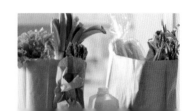

my numbers

weight _____   blood sugar (time/level) _____ / _____ • _____ / _____ • _____ / _____ • _____ / _____

what I ate today

circle the number of servings

fruit

0 1 2 3 **4**

vegetables

0 1 2 3 4 **5**

whole grains

0 1 2 3 4 5 **6**

calcium-rich foods

0 1 **2** **3**

beans

0 1 2

fish

0 1 2

extra lean poultry or meat

0 1 2

glasses of water

0 1 2 3 4 5 6 **7** **8** 9 10

times I ate out of boredom, stress, or habit

0 **1** 2 3 4 5

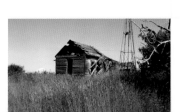

✳ **Tip of the day -** Be your own benchmark. Pay no attention to the next person's bulging biceps, trim waistline, or marathon medals. The exercise you're doing has nothing to do with anybody but you. Stay focused on your own goals, and don't compare yourself with others.

taking charge of my health!

eat

☐ ate a healthy breakfast
☐ had protein at every meal
☐ had 1-2 healthy snacks
☐ ate dinner by 7:00 p.m.
☐ avoided "white" foods
☐ drank water or tea instead of sugary drinks

move

☐ walked _____ steps/minutes
☐ made active choices
☐ got other exercise

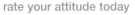

choose

☐ took my vitamins
☐ got enough sleep _____ hrs
☐ kept TV time under 2 hours

successes & confessions

rate your attitude today

3 excellent
2 good
1 so-so
0 disaster! plan to do better tomorrow

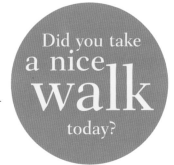

Did you take
a nice
walk
today?

saturday

my numbers

weight _____ blood sugar (time/level) _____ / _____ • _____ / _____ • _____ / _____ • _____ / _____

✳ **Tip of the day** - Cut down on alcohol. Beer, wine, and spirits are high in calories, and when you drink alcohol, you may be more likely to overeat the appetizers or order that indulgent, sugary dessert. If you want to enjoy a drink, choose a low-calorie beer or make a spritzer—a half glass of wine mixed with club soda.

taking charge of my health!

eat
☐ ate a healthy breakfast
☐ had protein at every meal
☐ had 1-2 healthy snacks
☐ ate dinner by 7:00 p.m.
☐ avoided "white" foods
☐ drank water or tea instead of sugary drinks

move
☐ walked _____ steps/minutes
☐ made active choices
☐ got other exercise
_____

choose
☐ took my vitamins
☐ got enough sleep _____ hrs
☐ kept TV time under 2 hours

successes & confessions

rate your attitude today
3 excellent
2 good
1 so-so
0 disaster! plan to do better tomorrow

Put your
fork
down
between bites
and eat more slowly.

what I ate today

circle the number of servings

fruit
0 1 2 3 **4**

vegetables
0 1 2 3 4 **5**

whole grains
0 1 2 3 4 5 **6**

calcium-rich foods
0 1 **2** 3

beans
0 1 2

fish
0 1 2

extra lean poultry or meat
0 1 2

glasses of water
0 1 2 3 4 5 6 **7** **8** 9 10

times I ate out of boredom, stress, or habit
0 **1** 2 3 4 5

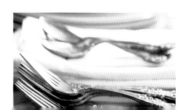

sunday

my numbers

weight _____   blood sugar (time/level) _____ / _____ • _____ / _____ • _____ / _____ • _____ / _____

what I ate today

circle the number of servings

fruit

0 1 2 3 **4**

vegetables

0 1 2 3 4 **5**

whole grains

0 1 2 3 4 5 **6**

calcium-rich foods

0 1 **2** **3**

beans

0 1 2

fish

0 1 2

extra lean poultry or meat

0 1 2

glasses of water

0 1 2 3 4 5 6 **7** **8** 9 10

times I ate out of boredom, stress, or habit

0 **1** 2 3 4 5

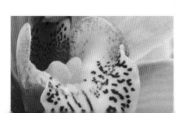

✳ **Tip of the day** - Save on fat—and time—by buying dry salad dressing mixes. Since you can control the amount of oil you add, you can use these mixes to create delicious, lower-fat dressings. Or sprinkle your salad with one tablespoon of olive oil and some flavorful vinegar, such as balsamic, or vinegars flavored with garlic, herbs, or spices. Limit yourself to one tablespoon of dressing.

taking charge of my health!

eat

☐ ate a healthy breakfast

☐ had protein at every meal

☐ had 1-2 healthy snacks

☐ ate dinner by 7:00 p.m.

☐ avoided "white" foods

☐ drank water or tea instead of sugary drinks

move

☐ walked _____ steps/minutes

☐ made active choices

☐ got other exercise

_____

choose

☐ took my vitamins

☐ got enough sleep _____ hrs

☐ kept TV time under 2 hours

successes & confessions

rate your attitude today

3   excellent

2   good

1   so-so

0   disaster! plan to do better tomorrow

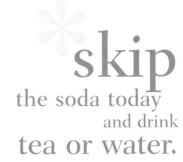

✳ **skip**
the soda today
and drink
tea or water.

week in review & ahead >

how well I did

eat

Improved my eating
from previous week   *[Yes] [No]*

Made healthy
restaurant choices   *[Yes] [No]*

Tried a new fruit,
vegetable, or grain   *[Yes] [No]*

move

Total walking time _____

Total steps _____
(if using a pedometer)

Walked more than
I did previous week   *[Yes] [No]*

Moved more than
I did previous week   *[Yes] [No]*

Felt more energized
than previous week   *[Yes] [No]*

choose

My attitude this week was:

☐ Positive—I can do this!

☐ Committed—I will follow
   through even if I falter here
   and there

☐ Defeated—need to
   remind myself that every
   little bit counts

Took time for myself   *[Yes] [No]*

Relaxed   *[Yes] [No]*

accomplishments!

_____
_____
_____
_____
_____
_____
_____
_____
_____
_____

☐ Weight loss? _____
☐ Waist measurement: _____
☐ Blood sugar improvement?
_____
_____

❝Never go to a
doctor whose office
plants have died.❞

—Erma Bombeck

next week's goals

eat Eat beans at least three
times next week. Add chickpeas
or kidney beans to salads. Add
white beans to pasta. Make
turkey or vegetarian chili. Make
a tasty black bean salad.

move Next week, you should
push your walks to 45 minutes—
your ultimate walking goal. If
you do, and you continue to walk
consistently, you'll slash your
risk of diabetes complications.

choose Next week, schedule any doctor's appointments
you're due for. Remember, if you
have diabetes, you should have
an eye exam every year and see
the dentist every six months.

✓ dms give us your feedback!

The diabetes management system is all about you. We created
it exclusively to help you take charge of your health and send
your blood sugar numbers down. So naturally, we want to hear
how you're doing! Write us at **dms@rd.com** and let us know
how much weight you've lost, whether your blood sugar has
dropped, and how your energy and attitude have improved as
a result of the changes you've made over the last 10 weeks.
Send us:

• Your success stories and personal anecdotes

• Healthy recipes you'd like to share

• Photos of the "new you"

• Your own tips and ideas for people with diabetes

• Feedback on the DMS

• Questions you'd like answered

• Other tools and products you'd like to have

We look forward to hearing from you!

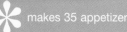

Cheesy Zucchini Bites

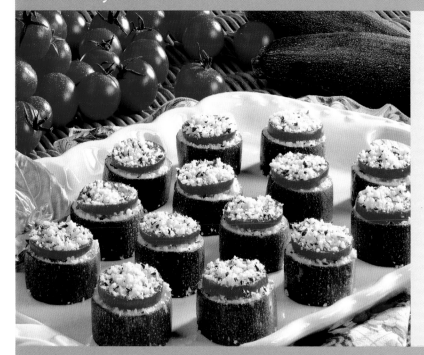

**Per serving
(one appetizer):**

19 calories
1 g fat
1 g saturated fat
3 mg cholesterol
58 mg sodium
1 g carbohydrate
0 fiber
1 g protein

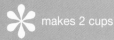
makes 2 cups

Asparagus Guacamole

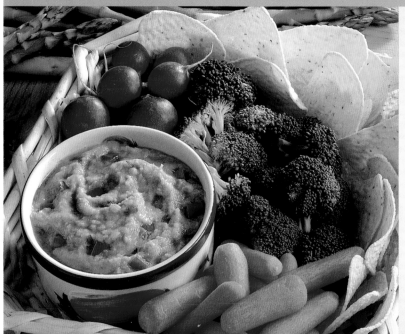

**Per serving
(1/3 cup guacamole):**

42 calories
2 g fat
0 g saturated fat
2 mg cholesterol
240 mg sodium
5 g carbohydrate
1 g fiber
3 g protein

5 medium zucchini (about 6 inches long)

4 ounces blue cheese, crumbled

3 tablespoons grated Parmesan cheese

1 teaspoon dried basil

1/8 teaspoon pepper

1 pint cherry tomatoes, thinly sliced

1. Cut zucchini into 3/4-inch slices. Using a melon baller or small spoon, scoop out the insides and discard, leaving the bottom intact. Place zucchini on an ungreased baking sheet; spoon 1/2 teaspoon crumbled blue cheese into each.

2. Combine the Parmesan cheese, basil, and pepper; sprinkle half over blue cheese. Top each with a tomato slice; sprinkle with the remaining Parmesan mixture. Bake at 400°F until cheese is melted, 5-7 minutes. Serve warm.

---

1 pound fresh asparagus, trimmed and cut into
   1-inch pieces

1/3 cup chopped onion

1 garlic clove

1/3 cup chopped seeded tomato

2 tablespoons reduced-fat mayonnaise

1 tablespoon lemon juice

1/2 teaspoon salt

3/4 teaspoon minced fresh cilantro or parsley

1/4 teaspoon chili powder

6 drops hot pepper sauce

Assorted raw vegetables and baked tortilla chips

1. Place 1/2 inch of water and asparagus in a saucepan; bring to a boil. Reduce heat; cover and simmer until tender, about 5 minutes. Drain; place asparagus in a blender or food processor. Add onion and garlic; cover and process until smooth.

2. In a bowl, combine tomato, mayonnaise, lemon juice, salt, cilantro, chili powder, and hot pepper sauce. Stir in the asparagus mixture until blended. Serve with vegetables and chips. Refrigerate leftovers; stir before serving.

Tomato Black Bean Salsa

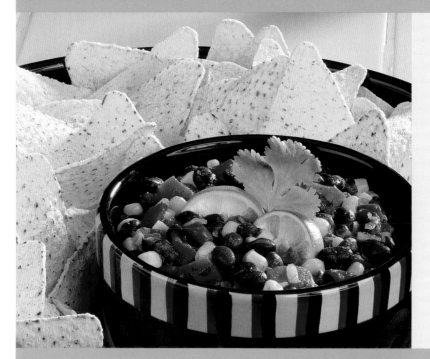

**Per serving
(1/2 cup salsa):**

80 calories
1 g fat
0 g saturated fat
0 mg cholesterol
318 mg sodium
15 g carbohydrate
4 g fiber
4 g protein

Raspberry-Beet-Berry Smoothie

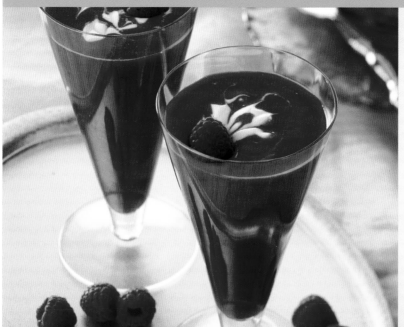

Per serving:

90 calories
1 g fat
1 g saturated fat
5 mg cholesterol
75 mg sodium
18 g carbohydrate
2 g fiber
4 g protein

3 medium tomatoes, seeded and chopped

1 can (15 ounces) black beans, rinsed and drained

3/4 cup fresh or frozen corn

1/2 cup finely chopped red onion

1/2 cup chopped roasted red pepper

1 jalapeño pepper, finely chopped*

2 tablespoons minced fresh cilantro or parsley

1/4 cup lime juice

1 garlic clove, minced

1 teaspoon dried oregano

1 teaspoon ground cumin

1/2 teaspoon salt

1/2 teaspoon ground coriander

Baked tortilla chips

In a large bowl, combine the first 13 ingredients. Cover and refrigerate for at least 2 hours before serving. Serve with tortilla chips.

*Editor's Note: When cutting or seeding hot peppers, use rubber or plastic gloves to protect your hands. Avoid touching your face.

2 cooked beets (4 1/2 ounces), cooled and coarsely chopped

2 ounces fresh or frozen raspberries

1 cup cranberry juice, chilled

1 cup low-fat plain yogurt

Chilled raspberries for garnish (optional)

1. In food processor or blender, puree beets, raspberries, and cranberry juice until smooth.

2. Pour puree through a strainer into a large pitcher. Whisk in most of the yogurt.

3. Pour into 4 glasses and top with remaining yogurt. Garnish with extra raspberries, if you like. Serve immediately.

Breakfast Burritos

serves 4

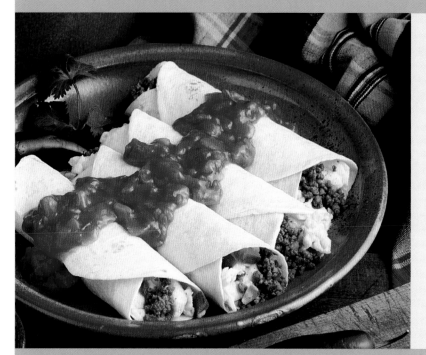

**Per serving
(without salsa):**

206 calories
3 g fat
2 g saturated fat
17 mg cholesterol
613 mg sodium
20 g carbohydrate
1 g fiber
23 g protein

Polish Apple Pancakes

serves 8

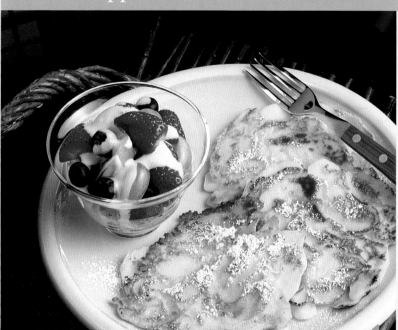

**Per serving
(2 pancakes):**

143 calories
3 g fat
1 g saturated fat
27 mg cholesterol
171 mg sodium
27 g carbohydrate
2 g fiber
4 g protein.

Egg substitute equivalent to 8 eggs

2 tablespoons finely chopped onion

2 tablespoons finely chopped green pepper

1 drop hot pepper sauce

1/2 cup shredded reduced-fat cheddar cheese

1/2 cup cooked taco-seasoned ground round

4 fat-free flour tortillas (6 inches), warmed

Salsa (optional)

1. In a bowl, combine egg substitute, onion, green pepper, hot pepper sauce, and cheese. Cook and stir in a nonstick skillet until eggs begin to set.

2. Add taco meat; cook until eggs are completely set.

3. Spoon onto a warmed tortilla and roll up; top with salsa if desired.

1 cup all-purpose flour

1 tablespoon sugar (optional)

1/2 teaspoon salt

1 egg

1 cup skim milk

1 tablespoon vegetable oil

5 medium apples, peeled and thinly sliced

Confectioners' sugar (optional)

1. In a bowl, combine flour, sugar if desired, and salt. In another bowl, lightly beat egg; add milk and oil. Add to dry ingredients and stir until smooth. Fold in apples.

2. Heat a griddle coated with nonstick cooking spray; pour batter by 1/2 cupfuls onto hot griddle and spread to form a 5-inch circle. Turn when bubbles begin to form on top. Cook until the second side is golden brown and apples are tender. Dust with confectioners' sugar if desired.

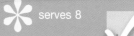

Fruit with Yogurt Sauce

serves 8

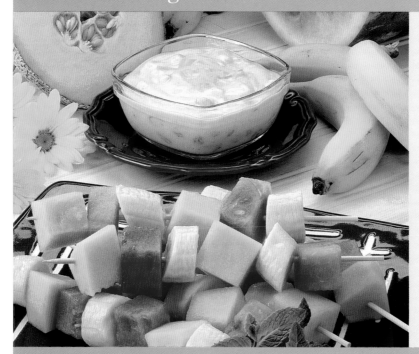

**Per serving
(with 2 tablespoons
sauce):**

170 calories
1 g fat
0 g saturated fat
1 mg cholesterol
47 mg sodium
40 g carbohydrate
3 g fiber
4 g protein

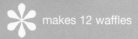

makes 12 waffles

Winter Squash Waffles

**Per serving
(one waffle):**

211 calories
7 g fat
1 g saturated fat
71 mg cholesterol
295 mg sodium
32 g carbohydrate
1 g fiber
5 g protein

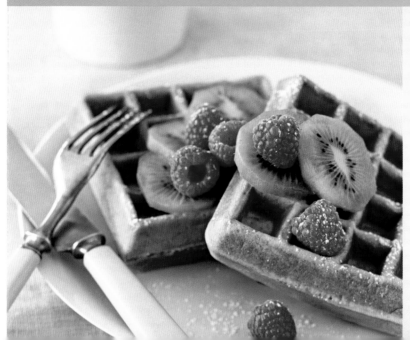

Yogurt Sauce

3/4 cup boiling water

1/4 cup raisins

1 carton (8 ounces) reduced-fat lemon yogurt

1/4 teaspoon ground ginger

1/8-1/4 teaspoon ground allspice

1/8-1/4 teaspoon ground cardamom

Fruit

4 large firm bananas, cut into 1/2-inch slices

2 tablespoons lemon juice

2 medium cantaloupe, peeled, seeded, and cubed

3 cups seeded, cubed watermelon

1. Place the water and raisins in a bowl; let stand for 5 minutes. Meanwhile, combine the yogurt, ginger, allspice, and cardamom in another bowl. Drain raisins; stir into yogurt mixture. Cover and refrigerate for at least 1 hour.

2. Toss bananas in lemon juice. Alternately thread fruit on wooden skewers or place in a serving bowl. Serve with yogurt sauce.

---

3 cups sifted cake flour

1 1/2 teaspoons baking soda

1 teaspoon cinnamon

1/2 teaspoon salt

4 large eggs

1/3 cup packed light-brown sugar

1 package (12 ounces) frozen pureed squash, thawed

3/4 cup low-fat buttermilk

1/4 cup vegetable oil

1 1/2 teaspoons grated orange zest

1 teaspoon vanilla extract

1. Preheat oven to 200°F. Preheat waffle iron.

2. In medium bowl stir together flour, baking soda, cinnamon, and salt. In large bowl stir together eggs and sugar. Stir in squash, buttermilk, oil, zest, and vanilla. Whisk in flour mixture just until smooth.

3. Lightly coat waffle iron with non-stick cooking spray. Pour batter, about 1/2 cup for each 4-inch-square waffle, onto iron, spreading quickly. Cook according to manufacturer's instructions. Place finished waffle on baking sheet in oven to keep warm. Make remaining waffles, coating waffle iron with cooking spray as needed. Serve hot with fresh fruit or hot maple syrup.

Creamy Greens Soup

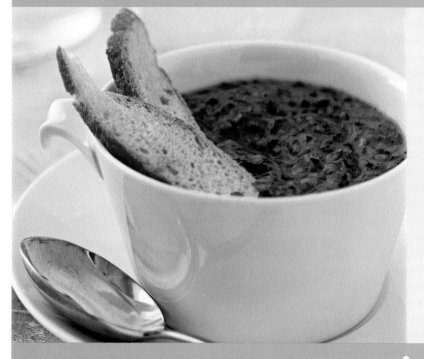

Per serving:

124 calories
4 g fat
2 g saturated fat
7 mg cholesterol
459 mg sodium
20 g carbohydrate
5 g fiber
5 g protein

Summer Garden Soup

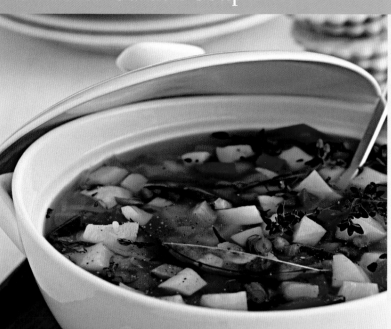

Per serving:

88 calories
2 g fat
0 g saturated fat
0 mg cholesterol
307 mg sodium
17 g carbohydrate
4 g fiber
3 g protein

2 teaspoons olive oil

2 leeks, pale green and white parts only, rinsed and coarsely chopped

1 medium onion, coarsely chopped

2 cloves garlic, minced

1 small bunch collard greens, stemmed and coarsely chopped

1 small bunch Swiss chard, stemmed and coarsely chopped

2 medium Yukon Gold or all-purpose potatoes, unpeeled and coarsely chopped

1 carrot, peeled and coarsely chopped

2 cans (14 1/2 ounces each) reduced-sodium, fat-free chicken broth

1 teaspoon salt

1/2 cup half-and-half

1. In large pot over medium heat, heat oil. Add leeks and onion. Sauté until softened, about 5 minutes. Add garlic; sauté 2 minutes. Add collard greens, Swiss chard, potatoes, and carrot. Stir in broth, 4 cups water, and salt. Simmer, partially covered, 50 minutes.

2. In blender or food processor, puree soup in small batches. Return to pot. Stir in half-and-half. Heat just until warmed through.

2 teaspoons olive oil

1 medium onion, finely chopped

1 large stalk celery, finely chopped

2 teaspoons finely chopped, peeled fresh ginger

1/4 pound green beans, cut into 1/2-inch pieces

2 medium potatoes, unpeeled and cut into 1/2-inch cubes

1 large carrot, peeled and cut into 1/2-inch cubes

1 medium yellow summer squash, quartered lengthwise, seeded, and cut into 1/2-inch cubes

1 bay leaf

3/4 teaspoon salt

3/4 cup fresh or frozen green peas

2 plum tomatoes, seeded and coarsely chopped

2 tablespoons finely chopped fresh basil leaves

1 1/2 teaspoons finely chopped fresh thyme leaves

1. In large pot over medium heat, heat oil. Add onion, celery, and ginger. Sauté until very tender, about 10 minutes. Add green beans, potatoes, carrot, squash, 8 cups water, bay leaf, and salt. Simmer, covered, 20 minutes.

2. Uncover soup. Simmer 15 minutes. For last 5 minutes, add peas, tomatoes, basil, and thyme. Remove bay leaf before serving.

serves 4

Greek Spinach, Egg and Lemon Soup

dms

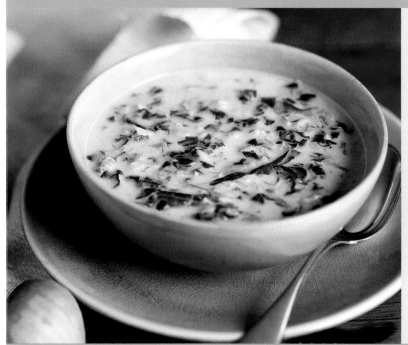

Per serving:

114 calories
2 g fat
1 g saturated fat
53 mg cholesterol
728 mg sodium
17 g carbohydrate
3 g fiber
8 g protein

serves 6

Chicken-Tomato Soup with Tortillas

dms

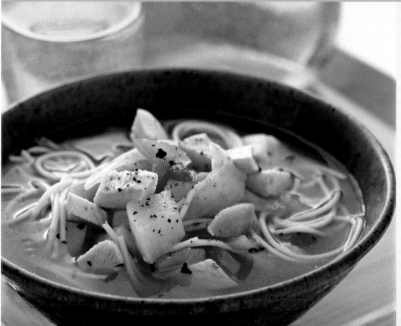

Per serving:

200 calories
5 g fat
1 g saturated fat
60 mg cholesterol
550 mg sodium
11 g carbohydrate
2 g fiber
25 g protein

3 cups reduced-sodium, fat-free chicken broth

3 scallions, thinly sliced

3 cloves garlic, minced

1 package (10 ounces) frozen chopped spinach

1/2 teaspoon oregano

1 cup cooked brown rice

1 teaspoon grated lemon zest

3 tablespoons fresh lemon juice

1/2 teaspoon salt

1 large egg plus 2 egg whites

1. In medium saucepan, combine 1/4 cup broth, scallions, and garlic. Cook over medium heat until scallions are tender, about 2 minutes.

2. Add remaining 2 3/4 cups broth, spinach, and oregano, and bring to a boil. Reduce to a simmer, cover, and cook until spinach is tender, about 5 minutes.

3. Stir in rice, lemon zest, lemon juice, and salt, and return to a simmer. Remove 1/2 cup hot liquid and whisk into whole egg and egg whites in medium bowl. Whisking constantly, pour warmed egg mixture into simmering soup.

---

1 whole bone-in chicken breast, skin removed

8 cups reduced-sodium, fat-free chicken broth

3 cloves garlic

1 teaspoon salt

1 teaspoon black pepper

1 teaspoon dried oregano, crumbled

1 tablespoon olive oil

5 scallions, coarsely chopped

1 can (4 1/2 ounces) green chiles, drained

4 medium tomatoes, coarsely chopped

1/2 cup fresh-squeezed lime juice

4 corn tortillas (6 inches), sliced into 3 x 1/4-inch strips, toasted

3 tablespoons chopped cilantro

1. Place chicken, broth, 2 cloves garlic, salt, pepper, and oregano in medium saucepan. Simmer, uncovered, 25 minutes.

2. Remove chicken from pot. Remove and discard bones. Cut chicken into large chunks. Strain and reserve broth.

3. In large saucepan over medium heat, heat oil. Mince remaining garlic. Add to saucepan along with scallions. Sauté until softened, 5 minutes. Add chiles, tomatoes, and strained broth. Simmer, partially covered, 15 minutes. (Recipe can be made ahead up to this point.)

4. Add chicken chunks, lime juice, and toasted tortilla strips. Simmer 5 minutes. Garnish with cilantro.

Turkey Spinach and Rice in Roasted Garlic Broth

 serves 4

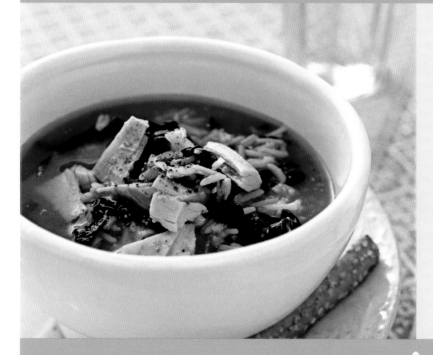

Per serving:

197 calories
4 g fat
1 g saturated fat
30 mg cholesterol
208 mg sodium
24 g carbohydrate
3 g fiber
19 g protein

Cabbage and Kielbasa Soup

 serves 6

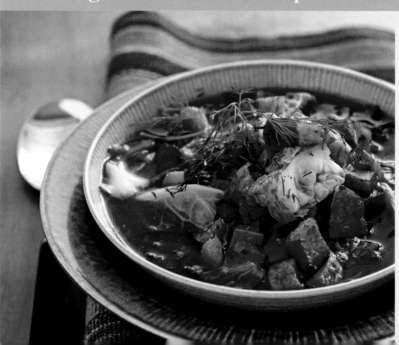

Per serving:

140 calories
3 g fat
0 g saturated fat
10 mg cholesterol
404 mg sodium
17 g carbohydrate
3 g fiber
10 g protein

2 medium whole heads garlic, unpeeled

2 tablespoons tomato paste

2 cans (14 1/2 ounces each) reduced-sodium, fat-free chicken or turkey broth

1 cup cooked turkey cubes

1 cup cooked long-grain white rice

3/4 pound spinach, stemmed and coarsely chopped

1/4 teaspoon black pepper

1/4 teaspoon hot pepper flakes, or to taste

1 tablespoon fresh-squeezed lemon juice

1. Preheat oven to 400°F.

2. Cut top third off garlic heads. Wrap each head in foil. Bake until very soft, about 50 minutes. Let cool. Remove foil. Squeeze out pulp into small bowl.

3. In large saucepan, stir together garlic pulp and tomato paste. Stir in broth. Bring to a boil. Add turkey, rice, spinach, pepper, and pepper flakes. Simmer, uncovered, 8 minutes. Just before serving, stir in lemon juice.

---

1 tablespoon vegetable oil

1/2 pound reduced-fat kielbasa sausage, diced

1 medium onion, coarsely chopped

4 cloves garlic, minced

2 cans (14 1/2 ounces each) reduced-sodium, fat-free beef broth

1 1/4 cups water

1/2 medium head Savoy cabbage, coarsely chopped (about 4 1/2 cups)

2 medium red potatoes, unpeeled, diced

2 medium carrots, peeled and diced

1 medium beet, peeled and diced

3 tablespoons finely chopped dill

1 bay leaf

1 tablespoon red-wine vinegar

1. In large saucepan over medium-high heat, heat oil. Add kielbasa. Sauté until browned, about 5 minutes. Add onion and garlic. Sauté until tender, about 5 minutes.

2. Add broth, water, cabbage, potatoes, carrots, beet, dill, and bay leaf. Simmer, covered, until vegetables are very tender, about 45 minutes. Stir in vinegar. Remove bay leaf and serve.

Cucumber, Radish and Snow Pea Salad

 serves 4

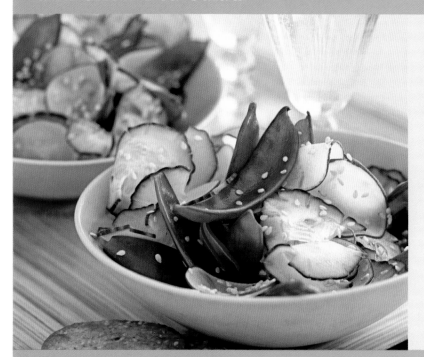

Per serving:

64 calories
2 g fat
0 g saturated fat
0 mg cholesterol
247 mg sodium
10 g carbohydrate
3 g fiber
3 g protein

 serves 8

Minty Fruit Salad

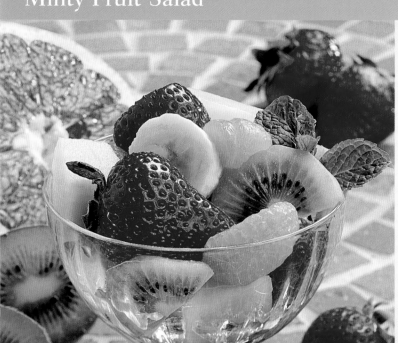

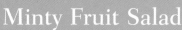

**Per serving
(1 cup):**

134 calories
0 g fat
0 g saturated fat
0 mg cholesterol
6 mg sodium,
34 g carbohydrate
3 g fiber
1 g protein

6 ounces snow peas, trimmed

1 tablespoon rice vinegar

2 teaspoons sugar

2 teaspoons soy sauce

1 teaspoon dark sesame oil

1/8 teaspoon salt

2 cucumbers, scored and thinly sliced

2 bunches radishes, thinly sliced

1 tablespoon sesame seeds, toasted *(optional)*

1. In saucepan of lightly salted boiling water, cook snow peas until crisp-tender, 2-3 minutes. Drain. Rinse under cold running water.

2. In small bowl, whisk together vinegar, sugar, soy sauce, sesame oil, and salt until sugar and salt are dissolved to make vinaigrette.

3. In large bowl, toss together snow peas, cucumbers, radishes, and vinaigrette. Sprinkle with sesame seeds, if using.

2 cups cubed honeydew

2 cups halved unsweetened strawberries

1 cup sliced banana

1 cup grapefruit segments

1 cup sliced halved peeled kiwifruit

1 cup mandarin oranges

1/2 cup sugar

1/3 cup orange juice

1/3 cup lemon juice

1/8 teaspoon peppermint extract

In a large bowl, combine the fruit. In a small bowl, combine the remaining ingredients. Pour over fruit and gently stir to coat. Cover and refrigerate for at least 3 hours.

Two-Cabbage Slaw

serves 6

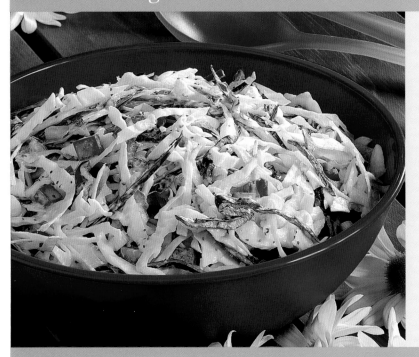

**Per serving
(1 cup):**

140 calories
4 g fat
3 g saturated fat
13 mg cholesterol
465 mg sodium
21 g carbohydrate
6 g fiber
6 g protein

serves 12

Garlic Green and Wax Beans

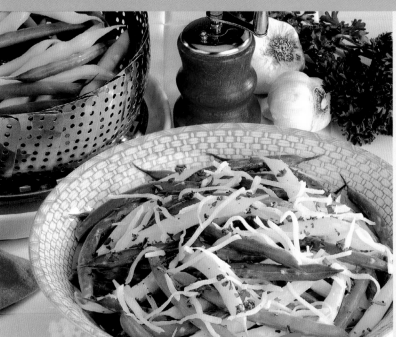

**Per serving
(3/4 cup):**

76 calories
2 g fat
1 g saturated fat
7 mg cholesterol
157 mg sodium
9 g carbohydrate
4 g fiber
5 g protein

Slaw

4 cups shredded green cabbage

1 cup shredded red cabbage

1 medium green pepper, chopped

1 medium sweet red pepper, chopped

4 scallions, finely chopped

Dressing

1 cup (8 ounces) reduced-fat sour cream

3 tablespoons tarragon vinegar or cider vinegar

1 tablespoon sugar

1 teaspoon salt

3/4 teaspoon celery seed

1/4 teaspoon white pepper

In a large bowl, combine the first five ingredients. In a small bowl, combine the dressing ingredients. Pour over cabbage mixture and stir to coat. Serve immediately.

---

1 1/2 pounds fresh green beans

1 1/2 pounds fresh wax beans

7 garlic cloves, minced, divided

1/4 cup reduced-fat sour cream

1/4 cup fat-free milk

1 teaspoon white wine vinegar or cider vinegar

1 teaspoon olive or canola oil

1/2 teaspoon salt

1/8 teaspoon pepper

1 cup shredded part-skim mozzarella cheese

Minced fresh parsley

1. In a large saucepan, place beans and six garlic cloves in a steamer basket over 1 inch of boiling water. Cover and steam until beans are crisp-tender, 8-10 minutes. Transfer to a large bowl; set aside.

2. In a small bowl, combine sour cream, milk, and vinegar; let stand for 1 minute. Whisk in the oil, salt, pepper, and remaining garlic. Pour over beans and toss.

3. Cover and chill for at least 2 hours. Just before serving, sprinkle with cheese and parsley.

Corn Relish Salad

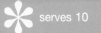

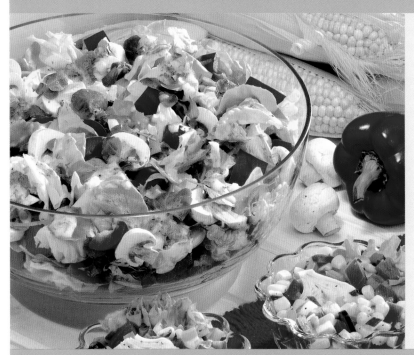

**Per serving
(3/4 cup):**

68 calories
2 g fat
0 g saturated fat
0 mg cholesterol
193 mg sodium
13 g carbohydrate
2 g fiber
2 g protein

Black-Eyed Pea Salad

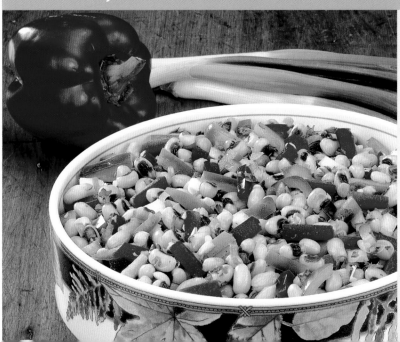

**Per serving
(3/4 cup):**

141 calories
1 g fat
0 g saturated fat
1 mg cholesterol
392 mg sodium
26 g carbohydrate
7 g fiber
8 g protein

2 cups fresh or frozen corn

3 medium tomatoes, seeded and chopped

1 medium green pepper, diced

1/2 cup chopped red onion

1/2 cup sliced celery

1 can (2 1/4 ounces) sliced ripe olives, drained

1 jar (6 1/2 ounces) marinated artichoke hearts, undrained

1/4 cup reduced-fat Italian salad dressing

5 fresh basil leaves, finely chopped or 1 teaspoon dried basil

1/2 teaspoon garlic powder

1/2 teaspoon dried oregano

1/4 teaspoon lemon-pepper seasoning

1. In a large bowl, combine the first six ingredients.

2. In another bowl, combine the artichokes, salad dressing, basil, garlic powder, oregano, and lemon-pepper. Add to corn mixture and toss gently.

3. Cover and refrigerate for at least 6 hours before serving.

---

1 pound dry black-eyed peas

1 cup fat-free Italian salad dressing

1/2 cup chopped onion

2 cups chopped green pepper

1 cup chopped sweet red pepper

3/4 cup finely chopped scallions

1/2 cup finely chopped seeded jalapeño peppers*

1/4 cup minced fresh parsley

3 garlic cloves, minced

1/2 teaspoon salt

1/8 teaspoon hot pepper sauce

1. Place peas in a Dutch oven or soup kettle; add water to cover by 2 inches. Bring to a boil; boil for 2 minutes. Remove from the heat; cover and let stand for 1 hour. Drain and rinse peas, discarding liquid. Return peas to pan; cover with water. Bring to a boil. Reduce heat; cover, and simmer until tender, about 1 hour.

2. Drain peas and place in a large bowl. Add salad dressing and onion; toss to coat. Cover and refrigerate until cool. Add the remaining ingredients; toss gently.

Editor's Note: When cutting or seeding hot peppers, use rubber or plastic gloves to protect your hands. Avoid touching your face.

Broccoli with Orange Sauce

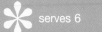

serves 6

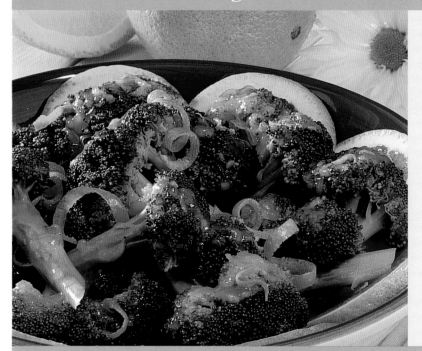

Per serving:

54 calories
0 g fat
0 g saturated fat
0 mg cholesterol
108 mg sodium
13 g carbohydrate
3 g fiber
3 g protein

Tex-Mex Corn on the Cob

serves 12

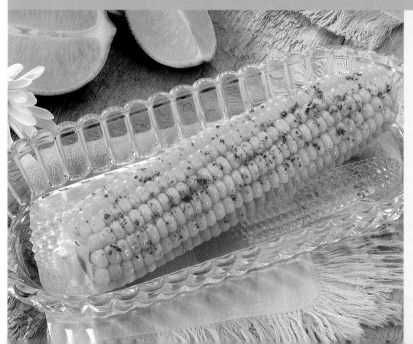

**Per serving
(1 ear):**

85 calories
1 g fat
0 g saturated fat
0 mg cholesterol
164 mg sodium
20 g carbohydrate
2 g fiber
3 g protein

1 pound fresh or frozen broccoli spears

4 1/2 teaspoons sugar

2 teaspoons cornstarch

1/2 teaspoon chicken bouillon granules

1/4 cup water

1/4 cup orange juice

1 teaspoon grated orange peel

1 medium navel orange, thinly sliced

1. Place broccoli and a small amount of water in a saucepan; bring to a boil. Reduce heat; cover and cook until crisp-tender, 5-8 minutes. Meanwhile, in a small saucepan, combine the sugar, cornstarch, and bouillon. Stir in water, orange juice, and peel until blended. Bring to a boil; cook and stir until thickened, about 2 minutes.

2. Drain broccoli and place in a serving bowl. Garnish with orange slices and drizzle with sauce .

12 small ears fresh corn on the cob (about 6 inches)

3 tablespoons minced fresh cilantro or parsley

1 1/2 teaspoons chili powder

1 1/2 teaspoons grated lime peel

3/4 teaspoon salt

3/4 teaspoon ground cumin

1/4 teaspoon garlic powder

Refrigerated butter-flavored spray.

1. Place corn in a Dutch oven or kettle; cover with water. Bring to a boil; cook until tender, 3-5 minutes. Meanwhile, in a small bowl, combine the cilantro, chili powder, lime peel, salt, cumin, and garlic powder.

2. Drain the corn. Spritz with butter-flavored spray; brush or pat seasonings over corn.

Zippy Green Beans

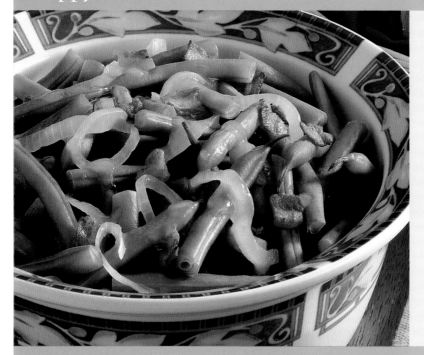

Per serving (3/4 cup):

98 calories
2 g fat
1 g saturated fat
3 mg cholesterol
140 mg sodium
16 g carbohydrate
3 g fiber
2 g protein

Stir-Fried Bok Choy with Sugar Snap Peas

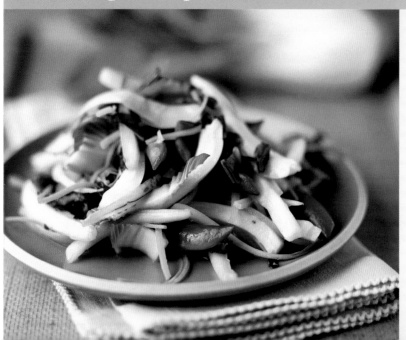

Per serving:

109 calories
3 g fat
1 g saturated fat
0 mg cholesterol
630 mg sodium
19 g carbohydrate
3 g fiber
4 g protein

4 cups fresh or frozen green beans, cut into
  2-inch pieces

2 bacon strips, diced

1 medium onion, thinly sliced

1/2 cup white wine or apple juice

3 tablespoons sugar

3 tablespoons tarragon vinegar or cider vinegar

1/4 teaspoon salt

2 teaspoons cornstarch

1 tablespoon cold water

1. Place beans in a saucepan and cover with water; bring to a boil. Cook, uncovered, until crisp-tender, 8-10 minutes. Meanwhile, in a large nonstick skillet, cook bacon over medium heat until crisp. Remove with a slotted spoon to paper towels. Drain, reserving 1 teaspoon drippings.

2. In the drippings, sauté onion until tender. Add wine or apple juice, sugar, vinegar, and salt. Combine cornstarch and cold water until smooth; add to the skillet. Bring to a boil; cook and stir until thickened, about 2 minutes. Drain beans; top with onion mixture. Sprinkle with bacon; toss to coat.

2 teaspoons olive oil

1 carrot, cut into matchsticks

2 tablespoons slivered fresh ginger

1 pound bok choy, cut into 1/2-inch-wide slices

8 ounces sugar snap peas, trimmed

3 tablespoons orange juice concentrate

1 tablespoon light-brown sugar

1 tablespoon reduced-sodium soy sauce

1/2 teaspoon salt

1 teaspoon cornstarch blended with
  1 tablespoon water

1. In large nonstick skillet over medium heat, heat 1/4 cup water and oil. Add carrot and ginger, and cook, stirring frequently, until carrot is crisp-tender, about 3 minutes.

2. Add bok choy, sugar snap peas, orange juice concentrate, brown sugar, soy sauce, and salt. Cover and cook until bok choy begins to wilt, about 3 minutes.

3. Uncover and cook, stirring frequently, until bok choy is crisp-tender, about 2 minutes. Stir in cornstarch mixture and cook, stirring constantly, until vegetables are evenly coated, about 1 minute.

Braised Cabbage with Apple and Caraway

 serves 6

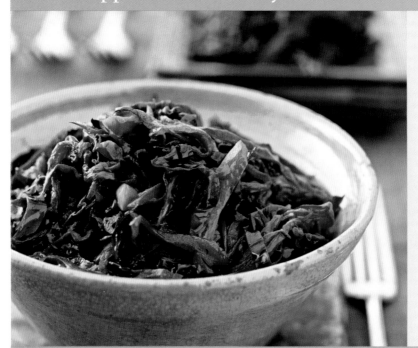

Per serving:

67 calories
2 g fat
0 g saturated fat
0 mg cholesterol
212 mg sodium
13 g carbohydrate
4 g fiber
2 g protein

 serves 6

Roasted Carrots with Rosemary

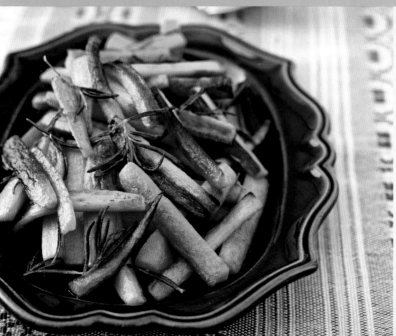

Per serving:

44 calories
1 g fat
0 g saturated fat
0 mg cholesterol
136 mg sodium
8 g carbohydrate
2 g fiber
1 g protein

2 teaspoons vegetable oil

1 small onion, finely chopped

3/4 teaspoon caraway seeds

1 pound green cabbage, cored and thinly sliced
(6 1/2 cups)

1 tablespoon rice wine vinegar or cider vinegar

1/2 teaspoon salt

2 small crisp red apples such as Gala, Braeburn,
or Empire, cored and cut into small cubes

1 teaspoon honey

2 tablespoons chopped walnuts,
toasted *(optional)*

1. Heat oil in large nonstick skillet over medium heat. Add onion and caraway seeds. Sauté until onion is softened, about 5 minutes.

2. Stir in cabbage, vinegar, and salt. Cover. Cook just until cabbage wilts, about 4 minutes. Uncover. Increase heat to high. Add apples and honey. Cook, stirring frequently, until apples are crisp-tender and most of liquid cooks off, 4-6 minutes. Transfer to serving plate. Top with walnuts, if desired.

1 pound large carrots, peeled and cut into
2 x 1/4-inch sticks

1/4 teaspoon salt

1 1/2 teaspoons olive oil

1 teaspoon minced fresh rosemary leaves or
1/2 teaspoon dried, crumbled

1. Preheat oven to 400°F.

2. Mound carrot sticks on baking sheet. Sprinkle with salt and drizzle with oil. Gently toss. Spread out on sheet into single layer.

3. Roast 10 minutes. Stir in rosemary. Roast until crisp-tender and lightly browned in spots, 7-10 minutes.

Irish Mashed Potatoes with Cabbage and Leeks

 serves 8

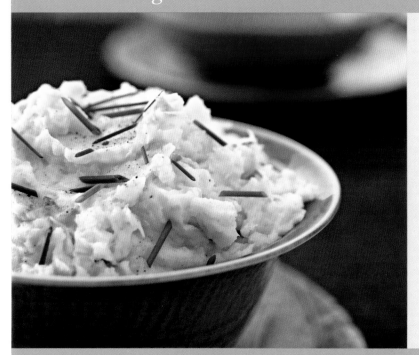

Per serving:

168 calories
4 g fat
2 g saturated fat
9 mg cholesterol
379 mg sodium
29 g carbohydrate
3 g fiber
6 g protein

Basmati Rice with Kale and Butternut Squash

 serves 6

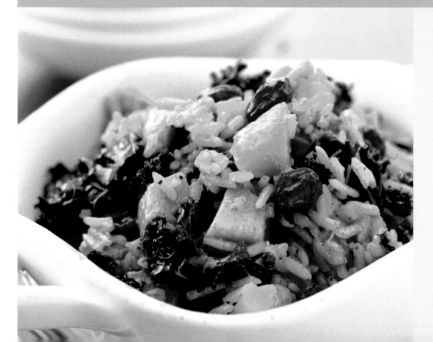

Per serving:

143 calories
3 g fat
1 g saturated fat
0 mg cholesterol
420 mg sodium
29 g carbohydrate
3 g fiber
4 g protein

2 pounds Yukon Gold potatoes, unpeeled and quartered

2 cans (14 1/2 ounces each) reduced-sodium, fat-free chicken broth

1 pound leeks, trimmed, thinly sliced, and rinsed

1 cup low-fat (1%) milk

3 cloves garlic, crushed

1 bay leaf

1 pound green cabbage, cored and thinly sliced

1/4 cup cold water

1/4 teaspoon ground nutmeg

1/4 teaspoon salt

1/4 teaspoon white pepper

2 tablespoons unsalted butter

1/4 cup minced chives

1. In large saucepan, combine potatoes, broth, and water as needed to cover potatoes with liquid. Boil potatoes until tender, 20-25 minutes.

2. Meanwhile, in second large saucepan, combine leeks, milk, garlic, and bay leaf. Cover. Bring to boil and simmer until leeks are softened, 15-20 minutes. Drain, reserving leeks, milk, and garlic separately. Discard bay leaf.

3. In same saucepan, combine cabbage and 1/4 cup water. Cover. Gently boil until tender, 10-15 minutes. Drain. Squeeze cabbage dry. Finely chop.

4. Drain potatoes and transfer to large bowl. Add milk and garlic to potatoes. Mash. Stir in leeks, cabbage, nutmeg, salt, pepper, and butter. Top with chives.

1/2 cup basmati rice

1 tablespoon curry powder

1 pound kale, tough stems removed and kale blanched

1/2 pound butternut squash, seeded, peeled, and cut in 3/4-inch pieces

1/4 cup raisins

1 cup reduced-fat coconut milk

3/4 cup water

1 teaspoon salt

1. Heat 12-inch nonstick skillet over medium-low heat. Add rice. Toast, stirring frequently, until lightly browned, about 3 minutes. Add curry powder. Cook, stirring, 1 minute.

2. Add kale, squash, raisins, coconut milk, water, and salt to skillet. Cover and simmer until liquid is absorbed and rice and squash are tender, about 12 minutes. Remove from heat. Let stand, covered, 5 minutes.

Sea Scallop and Cherry Tomato Sauté

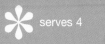 serves 4

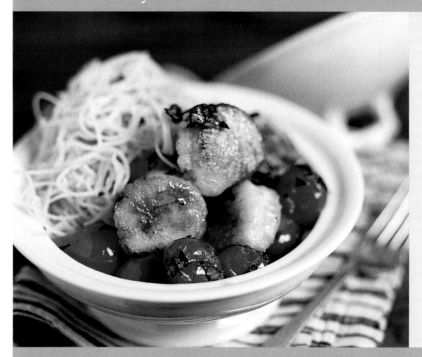

Per serving:

176 calories
4 g fat
1 g saturated fat
37 mg cholesterol
483 mg sodium
10 g carbohydrate
1 g fiber
20 g protein

Asian Steamed Fish Fillets with Vegetable Sticks

 serves 4

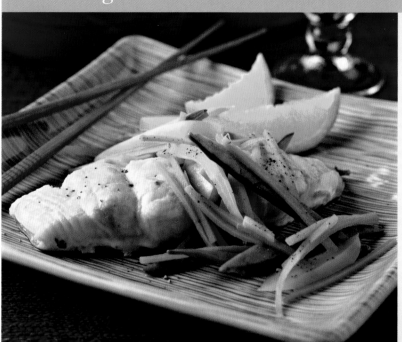

Per serving:

175 calories
3 g fat
0 g saturated fat
45 mg cholesterol
558 mg sodium
7 g carbohydrate
2 g fiber
32 g protein

1 pound sea scallops

4 teaspoons cornstarch

2 teaspoons olive oil

3 cloves garlic, minced

1 pint cherry tomatoes

2/3 cup dry vermouth, white wine,
   or chicken broth

1/2 teaspoon salt

1/3 cup chopped fresh basil

1 tablespoon cold water

1. Dredge scallops in 3 teaspoons cornstarch, shaking off excess. In large nonstick skillet over medium heat, heat oil. Add scallops and sauté until golden brown and cooked through, about 3 minutes. Transfer scallops to bowl.

2. Add garlic to pan and cook 1 minute. Add tomatoes and cook until they begin to collapse, about 4 minutes. Add vermouth, salt, and basil. Bring to a boil and cook 1 minute.

3. Stir together remaining 1 teaspoon cornstarch and cold water in small bowl. Add cornstarch mixture to pan and cook, stirring, until slightly thickened, about 1 minute.

4. Return scallops to pan. Simmer, and cook just until heated through, about 1 minute.

1 1/2 pounds halibut or other firm-fleshed white fish fillets, in 4 pieces

2 tablespoons soy sauce

2 tablespoons white wine or sake

1 thin slice fresh ginger, peeled and cut in thin sticks

2 medium carrots, peeled and cut into 3 x 1/4-inch sticks

2 ounces snow peas, cut in half lengthwise

1/2 yellow bell pepper, seeded and cut into thin sticks

1. Place fillets in baking dish that will fit inside large steamer basket or on rack that will fit into large skillet. In small cup, stir together soy sauce and white wine. Pour over fish. Top with ginger and carrots.

2. Fill skillet with 1 inch of water. Bring to a simmer. Place steamer basket or wire rack in skillet. Place baking dish containing fish in basket or on rack. Cover skillet or basket. Steam 5-6 minutes. Add snow peas and yellow pepper to baking dish. Cover. Steam until fish flakes when touched with fork and vegetables are crisp-tender, about 5 minutes. Serve at once.

Baked Cod Casserole
with Potatoes, Tomatoes and Arugula

serves 4

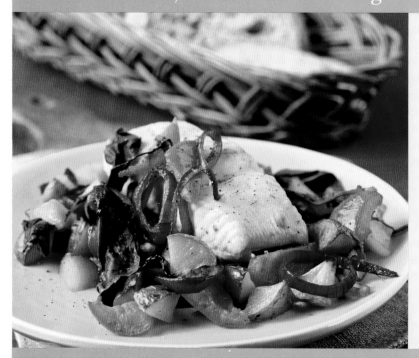

Per serving:

213 calories
5 g fat
1 g saturated fat
43 mg cholesterol
363 mg sodium
21 g carbohydrate
4 g fiber
22 g protein

 serves 6

Spicy Scallop Fettuccine

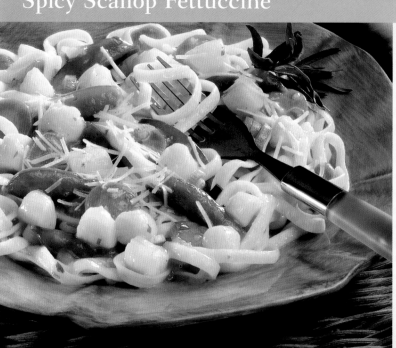

**Per serving
(1 cup):**

422 calories
10 g fat
4 g saturated fat
50 mg cholesterol
741 mg sodium
49 g carbohydrate
5 g fiber
30 g protein

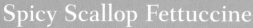

1 pound red potatoes, unpeeled and cut in 1/2-inch-thick slices

1 onion, thinly sliced

1 tablespoon olive oil

1/2 teaspoon salt

4 plum tomatoes, seeded and coarsely chopped

3 cloves garlic, minced

1/2 teaspoon dried oregano, crumbled

1 1/2 cups arugula leaves

1 pound cod, scrod, halibut, or other thick, firm-fleshed white fish steaks, cut into 2-inch chunks

1. Preheat oven to 350°F. In a 13 x 9 x 2-inch baking dish, combine potatoes, onion, oil, and 1/4 teaspoon salt.

2. Bake 20 minutes, stirring the mixture once.

3. Stir tomatoes, garlic, and oregano into potato mixture. Spread arugula on top in even layer. Top with cod. Sprinkle with remaining 1/4 tea-spoon salt.

4. Bake, covered with aluminum foil, just until fish is cooked through, 15-18 minutes. Transfer fish and vegetable mixture to serving plates. Spoon pan juices over each serving.

---

8 ounces uncooked fettuccine

2 large carrots, thinly sliced

1 tablespoon olive or canola oil

2 cups frozen sugar snap peas

3 scallions, sliced

3 garlic cloves, minced

1 tablespoon butter or stick margarine

1/2 cup white wine or chicken broth

1/3 cup water

2 teaspoons dried tarragon

1 teaspoon chicken bouillon granules

1/8-1/4 teaspoon cayenne pepper

1 pound fresh or frozen bay scallops, thawed

2 tablespoons cornstarch

2 tablespoons cold water

1/4 cup shredded Parmesan cheese

1. Cook fettuccine according to package directions. Meanwhile, in a large nonstick skillet, sauté carrots in oil for 4 minutes. Add the peas, scallions, and garlic; sauté until car-rots are tender, about 3 minutes. Remove vegetables and keep warm. Drain fettuccine and toss with butter; keep warm.

2. In the skillet, combine wine or broth, water, tarragon, bouillon, and cayenne. Bring to a boil; add scal-lops. Reduce heat; simmer, uncovered, for 1 minute. Combine cornstarch and cold water until smooth; stir into skillet. Bring to a boil; cook and stir until sauce is thickened and scallops are opaque, about 2 minutes. Add pasta and veg-etables; heat through. Sprinkle with Parmesan cheese.

Grilled Chicken Breast with Corn and Pepper Relish

serves 4

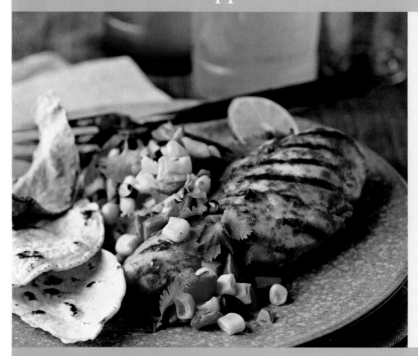

Per serving:

375 calories
12 g fat
2 g saturated fat
95 mg cholesterol
521 mg sodium
29 g carbohydrate
5 g fiber
40 g protein

Orange Turkey Stir-Fry

serves 4

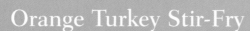
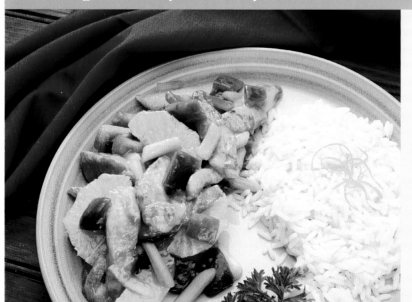

Per serving:

289 calories
4 g fat
1 g saturated fat
54 mg cholesterol
353 mg sodium
35 g carbohydrate
3 g fiber
30 g protein

2 cloves garlic, minced

2 teaspoons chili powder

1/4 teaspoon salt

3 tablespoons fresh-squeezed lime juice

2 tablespoons vegetable oil

1 1/2 pounds boneless, skinless chicken breasts, pounded 3/8 inch thick

3/4 cup reduced-sodium, fat-free chicken broth

1 1/2 cups fresh, drained canned, or thawed frozen corn kernels

1 cup diced, seeded, roasted red bell pepper

2/3 cup canned black beans, drained and rinsed

2 tablespoons coarsely chopped red onion

1 jalapeño pepper, seeded and finely chopped*

1/4 teaspoon salt

3 tablespoons chopped cilantro

1. In medium bowl, stir together garlic, chili powder, salt, 2 tablespoons lime juice, and oil. Add chicken and rub with marinade. Let stand no more than 15 minutes.

2. Preheat grill to medium-hot or preheat broiler. Grill or broil chicken 3 inches from heat just until cooked through, 3-4 minutes per side.

3. To make relish: In large skillet, heat broth. Add corn kernels, bell pepper, black beans, onion, chile, and salt. Heat through. Stir in cilantro and remaining lime juice, and serve chicken topped with relish.

Editor's Note: When cutting or seeding hot peppers, use rubber or plastic gloves to protect your hands. Avoid touching your face.

3/4 cup orange juice

1/4 cup orange marmalade

2 tablespoons light soy sauce

2 tablespoons cornstarch

1/8 teaspoon ground ginger

1/8 teaspoon hot pepper sauce

1 pound turkey tenderloin, trimmed and cut into 1-inch strips

1/4 cup all-purpose flour

2 teaspoons cooking oil

4 scallions, cut into 1-inch pieces

1/2 cup coarsely chopped green pepper

1 seedless orange, peeled, sliced and halved

Hot cooked rice *(optional)*

1. In a small bowl, combine the first six ingredients; set aside.

2. Dredge turkey in flour; shake off excess. In a 10-inch skillet, heat oil over medium-high heat. Cook turkey in three batches until tender and lightly browned on all sides. Remove and keep warm.

3. Add scallions and green pepper to the skillet; cook and stir for 1 minute. Stir in orange juice mixture. Bring to a boil; reduce heat and simmer for 3 minutes. Add turkey and oranges; heat through. Serve over rice if desired.

Curry Chicken Dinner

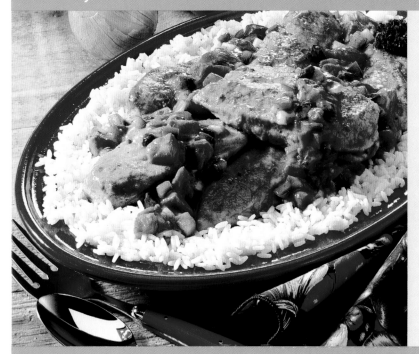

Per serving:

230 calories
6 g fat
1 g saturated fat
63 mg cholesterol
233 mg sodium
17 g carbohydrate
2 g fiber
25 g protein

Turkey Tetrazzini

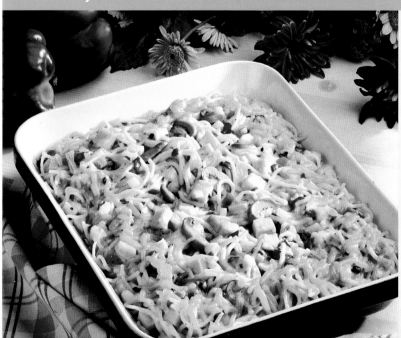

Per serving:

223 calories
6 g fat
3 g saturated fat
28 mg cholesterol
288 mg sodium
26 g carbohydrate
2 g fiber
16 g protein

8 boneless, skinless chicken breast halves
(2 pounds)

1/2 cup all-purpose flour

2 tablespoons cooking oil

2 medium onions, chopped

2 medium green peppers, chopped

1 garlic clove, minced

2 teaspoons curry powder

1/2 teaspoon white pepper

2 cans (14 1/2 ounces each) diced tomatoes,
undrained

1 teaspoon chopped fresh parsley

1/2 teaspoon dried thyme

1 cup water

3 tablespoons raisins

Hot cooked rice *(optional)*

1. Dust chicken with flour. In a Dutch oven over medium heat, brown the chicken in oil. Remove chicken and set aside.

2. Add onions, green peppers, and garlic to drippings; sauté until tender, 3-4 minutes. Add curry and pepper; mix well. Return chicken to the pan. Add tomatoes, parsley, thyme, and water.

3. Cover and bake at 375°F until chicken is tender and juices run clear, 45-50 minutes. Stir in raisins. Serve over rice if desired.

1 package (7 ounces) spaghetti, broken into 2-inch pieces

2 cups cubed, cooked turkey breast

1 cup (4 ounces) shredded reduced-fat cheddar cheese

1 can (10 3/4 ounces) low-fat condensed cream of mushroom soup, undiluted

1 medium onion, chopped

2 cans (4 ounces each) sliced mushrooms, drained

1/3 cup skim milk

1/4 cup chopped green pepper

1 jar (2 ounces) diced pimientos, drained

1/8 teaspoon pepper

Additional shredded reduced-fat cheddar cheese *(optional)*

Cook spaghetti according to package directions; drain. Transfer to a large bowl; add the next nine ingredients and mix well. Spoon into a 2 1/2-quart casserole coated with nonstick cooking spray; sprinkle with cheese if desired. Bake, uncovered, at 375°F until heated through, 40-45 minutes.

Pepper-Topped Beef Sandwiches

serves 6

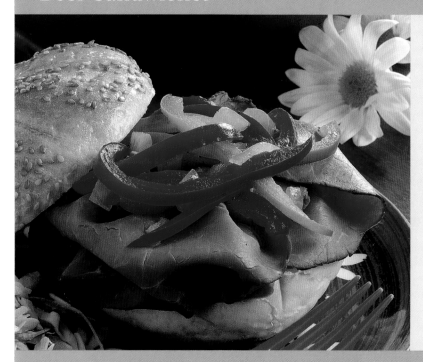

Per serving:

325 calories
8 g fat
2 g saturated fat
46 mg cholesterol
568 mg sodium
39 g carbohydrate
3 g fiber
23 g protein

makes 2 pizzas

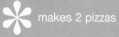

South-of-the-Border Pizza

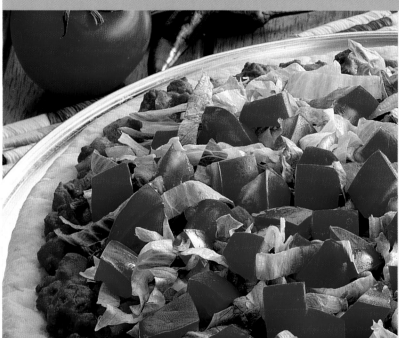

**Per serving
(one slice):**

250 calories
7 g fat
3 g saturated fat
20 mg cholesterol
706 mg sodium
31 g carbohydrate
5 g fiber
17 g protein

1 medium onion, chopped

2 garlic cloves, minced

1 tablespoon olive or canola oil

1 medium sweet red pepper, julienned

1 medium green pepper, julienned

1 bay leaf

1/2 teaspoon salt

1/8 teaspoon pepper

1 tablespoon sugar

12 ounces thinly sliced deli roast beef

6 sandwich rolls, split

In a nonstick skillet, sauté onion and garlic in oil until tender. Add the red and green peppers, bay leaf, salt, and pepper. Cook and stir until peppers are tender, about 10 minutes. Add sugar; cover and simmer until flavors are blended, 10-15 minutes. Discard bay leaf. Place beef on rolls; top with pepper mixture.

1 tablespoon cornmeal

1 loaf (1 pound) frozen bread dough, thawed

1/2 pound lean ground beef

1 medium onion, chopped

1 sweet yellow pepper, chopped

1 garlic clove, minced

1 can (16 ounces) fat-free refried beans

1 cup salsa

1 can (4 ounces) chopped green chiles

1-2 teaspoons chili powder

2 cups (8 ounces) shredded reduced-fat Mexican-blend cheese

2 medium tomatoes, chopped

2 cups shredded lettuce

1. Coat two 12-inch pizza pans with nonstick cooking spray; sprinkle with cornmeal. Divide the bread dough in half; roll each portion into a 12-inch circle. Transfer to prepared pans. Build up edges slightly; prick dough thoroughly with a fork. Bake at 425°F until lightly browned, about 12 minutes.

2. Meanwhile, in a skillet, cook the beef, onion, yellow pepper, and garlic over medium heat until meat is no longer pink; drain. Stir in refried beans, salsa, chiles, and chili powder; heat through. Spread over the crusts; sprinkle with cheese.

3. Bake until cheese is melted, 6-7 minutes. Top with tomatoes and lettuce; serve immediately.

Pork Chop Veggie Medley

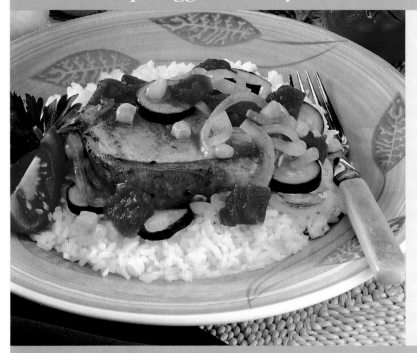

**Per serving
(1 chop and 1 cup
vegetable mixture
with 2/3 cup rice):**

418 calories
9 g fat
3 g saturated fat
62 mg cholesterol
455 mg sodium
52 g carbohydrate
5 g fiber
32 g protein

Honey-Lime Pork Chops

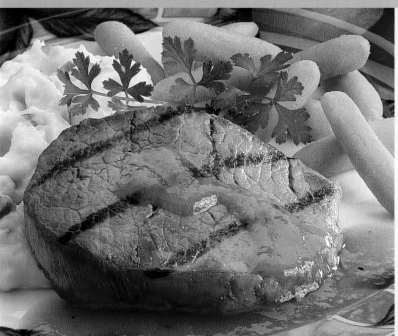

**Per serving
(1 chop with
2 tablespoons
sauce):**

200 calories
5 g fat
2 g saturated fat
71 mg cholesterol
884 mg sodium
11 g carbohydrate
0 g fiber
26 g protein

2 medium onions, thinly sliced

2 garlic cloves, minced

1 tablespoon olive or canola oil

6 boneless pork loin chops (3/4 inch thick and 4 ounces each)

1/2 teaspoon salt

1/4 teaspoon pepper

1/3 cup water

1 can (28 ounces) diced tomatoes, undrained

1 package (10 ounces) frozen corn

3 small zucchini, thinly sliced

4 cups hot cooked rice

1. In a large nonstick skillet, sauté onions and garlic in oil for 2-3 minutes. Add the pork chops; brown on both sides and sprinkle with salt and pepper. Remove chops and onions with a slotted spoon; keep warm.

2. Add water to drippings; bring to a boil, scraping any browned bits from pan. Return chops and onions to pan; add the tomatoes. Bring to a boil. Reduce heat; cover and simmer until meat is tender, 25-30 minutes.

3. Stir in corn and zucchini; cover and simmer until the vegetables are tender, 10-15 minutes. Serve over rice.

Chops

1/2 cup lime juice

1/2 cup reduced-sodium soy sauce

2 tablespoons honey

2 garlic cloves, minced

6 boneless pork loin chops (4 ounces each)

Sauce

3/4 cup reduced-sodium chicken broth

1 garlic clove, minced

1 1/2 teaspoons honey

1/2 teaspoon lime juice

1/8 teaspoon browning sauce

Dash pepper

2 teaspoons cornstarch

2 tablespoons water

1. In a large resealable plastic bag, combine the lime juice, soy sauce, honey, and garlic. Add pork chops. Seal bag and turn to coat; refrigerate for 8 hours or overnight. Drain and discard marinade. Grill chops, covered, over medium heat or broil 4 inches from the heat until juices run clear, 6-7 minutes on each side.

2. For sauce, combine the broth, garlic, honey, lime juice, browning sauce, and pepper in a small saucepan. Bring to a boil. Combine the cornstarch and water until smooth; stir into the broth mixture. Return to a boil; cook and stir until thickened, 1-2 minutes. Serve with the pork chops.

Chili with White Beans, Tomatoes and Corn

  serves 6

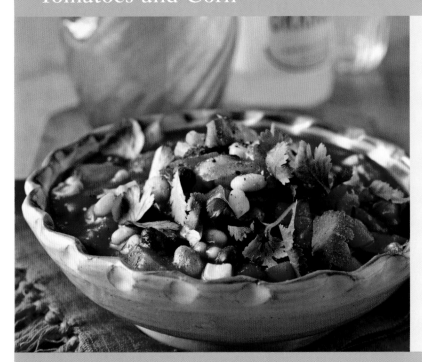

Per serving:

274 calories
7 g fat
1 g saturated fat
0 mg cholesterol
856 mg sodium
48 g carbohydrate
13 g fiber
15 g protein

Barley Risotto with Asparagus and Mushrooms

  serves 4

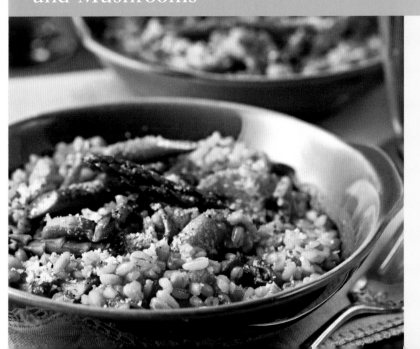

Per serving:

329 calories
10 g fat
2 g saturated fat
23 mg cholesterol
743 mg sodium
49 g carbohydrate
10 g fiber
15 g protein

2 tablespoons vegetable oil

1 large onion, finely chopped

1 red bell pepper, seeded and coarsely chopped

1 small carrot, peeled and diced

1 small celery stalk, diced

4 cloves garlic, minced

3 tablespoons chili powder

2 tablespoons sweet paprika

2 teaspoons dried oregano, crumbled

1 teaspoon ground cumin

1 can (28 ounces) whole tomatoes with their liquid, chopped

2 cans (19 ounces each) cannellini beans, drained and rinsed

1 can (15 ounces) black beans, drained and rinsed

1 cup water

1/4 cup reduced-sodium soy sauce

1 box (10 ounces) corn kernels

1. In large nonstick saucepan over medium-high heat, heat oil. Add onion, bell pepper, carrot, celery, and garlic. Cook until vegetables are softened, about 5 minutes. Stir in chili powder, paprika, oregano, and cumin. Cook 1 minute.

2. Add tomatoes, beans, water, and soy sauce to saucepan. Simmer, uncovered, 30 minutes, stirring occasionally. Stir in corn. Simmer 10 minutes more.

2 cans (14 1/2 ounces each) reduced-sodium, fat-free chicken broth

2 tablespoons olive oil

1 onion, finely chopped

8 ounces mushrooms, preferably mixture of wild varieties, coarsely chopped

2 cloves garlic, minced

1 cup pearl barley

8 ounces asparagus, trimmed, and cut into bite-size pieces, leaving tips whole

1/2 cup grated Parmesan cheese

1. In medium saucepan, heat broth and 2 cups water to just below a simmer. Cover; keep at a simmer.

2. In large deep nonstick skillet over medium heat, heat oil. Sauté onion about 3 minutes. Add mushrooms and garlic. Sauté until mushrooms are softened, about 5 minutes. Stir in barley. Stir in 2 cups hot broth mixture. Simmer, covered, 15 minutes.

3. Blanch asparagus tips in the pot of hot broth for 2 minutes. Transfer with slotted spoon to plate.

4. Add hot broth to barley mixture, 1/2 cup at a time, stirring. Let each batch of liquid be absorbed before adding more. When adding last batch of liquid, stir in asparagus stem pieces. Stir in Parmesan. Serve risotto topped with asparagus tips.

Homemade Pumpkin Spice Ice Cream

  serves 6

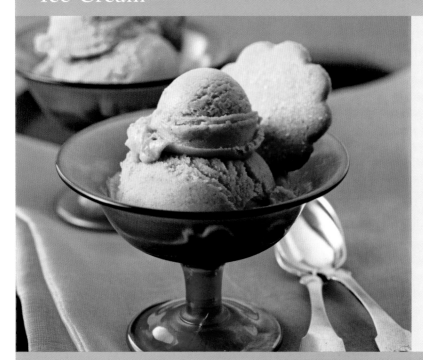

**Per serving
(1/2 cup):**

141 calories
1 g fat
1 g saturated fat
40 mg cholesterol
102 mg sodium
26 g carbohydrate
1 g fiber
5 g protein

Watermelon Ice

  serves 4

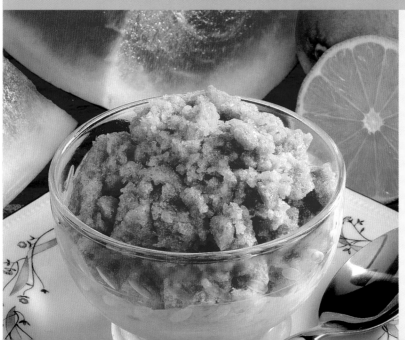

**Per serving
(3/4 cup):**

85 calories
1 g fat
0 g saturated fat
0 mg cholesterol
5 mg sodium
20 g carbohydrate
1 g fiber
2 g protein

1 1/4 cups evaporated low-fat (2%) milk

1 large egg

1/2 cup packed light-brown sugar

2/3 cup canned solid-pack pumpkin puree

1 teaspoon vanilla extract

1/2 teaspoon ground ginger

1/2 teaspoon cinnamon

Large pinch ground nutmeg

Pinch salt

1. In medium saucepan, bring milk to a boil.

2. In large bowl, whisk together egg and sugar. Gradually whisk in boiling milk. Stir in pumpkin, vanilla, ginger, cinnamon, nutmeg, and salt. Refrigerate until thoroughly chilled.

3. Freeze in ice-cream maker, following manufacturer's directions. Soften slightly before serving.

1 teaspoon unflavored gelatin

2 tablespoons water

4 cups seeded, cubed watermelon, divided

2 tablespoons lime juice

2 tablespoons honey

1. In a microwave-safe bowl, sprinkle gelatin over water; let stand for 2 minutes. Microwave on High for 40 seconds; stir. Let stand until gelatin is dissolved, about 2 minutes. Pour into a blender or food processor; add 1 cup watermelon, lime juice, and honey. Cover and process until smooth. Add remaining melon, a cup at a time, and process until smooth.

2. Pour into a 9-inch square dish; freeze until almost firm. Transfer to a chilled bowl; beat with an electric mixer until mixture is bright pink. Pour into serving dishes; freeze until firm. Remove from the freezer 15-20 minutes before serving.

Sunny Sponge Cake

serves 12

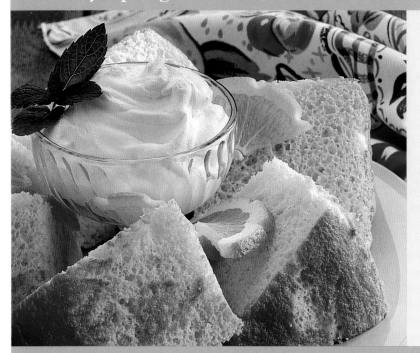

**Per serving
(1 slice with
1 tablespoon
whipped topping):**

160 calories
2 g fat
1 g saturated fat
53 mg cholesterol
103 mg sodium
31 g carbohydrate
0 g fiber
4 g protein

Ribbon Pudding Pie

serves 8

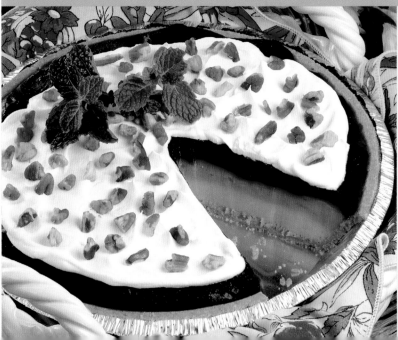

**Per serving
(1 slice):**

107 calories
2 g fat
1 g saturated fat
2 mg cholesterol
512 mg sodium
17 g carbohydrate
0 g fiber
5 g protein

3 egg yolks

1 cup sugar, divided

2 teaspoons hot water

1/2 cup orange juice, warmed

1 1/4 teaspoons vanilla extract

3/4 teaspoon grated orange peel

1/4 teaspoon grated lemon peel

1 1/2 cups all-purpose flour

1 1/4 teaspoons baking powder

1/4 teaspoon salt

6 egg whites

3/4 cup reduced-fat whipped topping

1. In a mixing bowl, beat egg yolks until slightly thickened. Gradually add 3/4 cup sugar and hot water, beating until thick and lemon-colored. Blend in the orange juice, vanilla, and orange and lemon peels. Sift together the flour, baking powder, and salt; add to egg yolk mixture.

2. In another mixing bowl, beat the egg whites until soft peaks form. Add the remaining sugar, 1 tablespoon at a time, beating until stiff peaks form. Fold a fourth of the egg whites into the batter; fold in remaining whites.

3. Spoon into an ungreased 10-inch tube pan. Bake at 350°F until cake springs back when lightly touched, 20-25 minutes. Immediately invert pan; cool completely. Cut into slices; serve with whipped topping.

4 cups cold fat-free milk, divided

1 package (1 ounce) sugar-free instant vanilla pudding mix

1 reduced-fat graham cracker crust (8 inches)

1 package (1 ounce) sugar-free instant butterscotch pudding mix

1 package (1.4 ounces) sugar-free instant chocolate pudding mix

1/2 cup reduced-fat whipped topping

2 tablespoons chopped pecans

1. In a mixing bowl, beat 1 1/3 cups milk and vanilla pudding mix on low speed for 2 minutes. Pour into graham cracker crust.

2. In another bowl, beat 1 1/3 cups milk and butterscotch pudding mix for 2 minutes. Spoon evenly over the vanilla layer.

3. Beat chocolate pudding mix and remaining milk for 2 minutes. Spread evenly over butterscotch layer.

4. Spread with whipped topping. Sprinkle with pecans. Refrigerate for at least 30 minutes.

Cool Mandarin Dessert

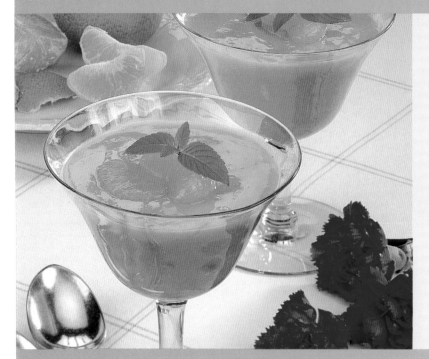

**Per serving
(1/2 cup):**

134 calories
1 g fat
0 g saturated fat
2 mg cholesterol
462 mg sodium
15 g carbohydrate
0 g fiber
7 g protein

Chocolate Pudding Sandwiches

 makes 43 sandwiches

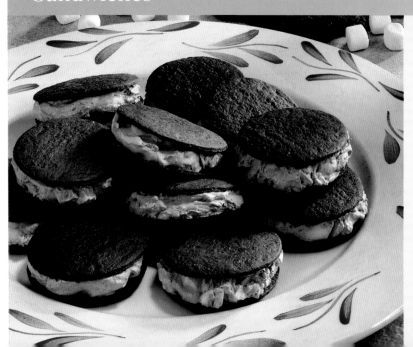

**Per serving
(one sandwich):**

73 calories
2 g fat
1 g saturated fat
1 mg cholesterol
114 mg sodium
12 g carbohydrate
0 g fiber
1 g protein

1 can (11 ounces) mandarin oranges

2 packages (.3 ounce each) sugar-free orange gelatin

2 cups boiling water

1 pint orange sherbet

Fresh mint (optional)

1. Drain oranges, reserving the juice; add enough water to juice to measure 1 cup. Refrigerate the oranges. In a large bowl, dissolve gelatin in boiling water. Stir in reserved juice. Add sherbet, stirring until dissolved. Refrigerate for 1 hour or until thickened.

2. Keep 10 orange segments refrigerated for garnish. Fold remaining oranges into gelatin mixture; cover and refrigerate overnight. Just before serving, garnish with reserved oranges and mint if desired.

1 1/2 cups cold fat-free milk

1 package (1.4 ounces) sugar-free instant chocolate pudding mix

1 carton (8 ounces) frozen reduced-fat whipped topping, thawed

1 cup miniature marshmallows

2 packages (9 ounces each) chocolate wafers

1. In a bowl, whisk milk and pudding mix until slightly thickened, about 2 minutes. Fold in whipped topping and marshmallows.

2. For each sandwich, spread about 2 tablespoons pudding mixture on a chocolate wafer; top with another wafer.

3. Stack sandwiches in an airtight container. Freeze until firm, about 3 hours. Remove from the freezer 5 minutes before serving.